What to do Between the Tears...

A Practical Guide to Dealing with a Dementia
or Alzheimer's Diagnosis in the Family

Feel less overwhelmed and more empowered.
You don't have to go through this alone...

by Tara Reed

This edition is published by Pivot to Happy Press,
a division of Pivot to Happy / Tara Reed Designs Inc

www.PivotToHappy.com/alz/

Tara Reed Designs Inc
11575 SW Pacific Hwy, #143
Tigard, Oregon 97223

ISBN-13: 978-0692567623

What to Do Between the Tears...

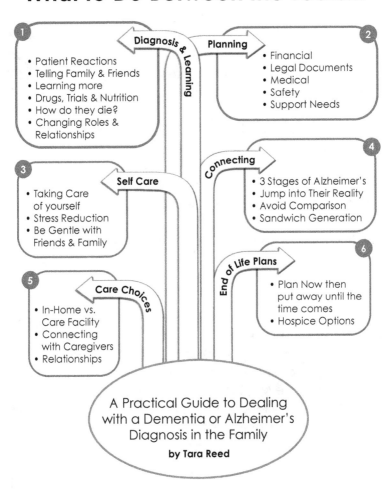

1

Diagnosis & Learning

- Patient Reactions
- Telling Family & Friends
- Learning more
- Drugs, Trials & Nutrition
- How do they die?
- Changing Roles & Relationships

2

Planning

- Financial
- Legal Documents
- Medical
- Safety
- Support Needs

3

Self Care

- Taking Care of yourself
- Stress Reduction
- Be Gentle with Friends & Family

4

Connecting

- 3 Stages of Alzheimer's
- Jump into Their Reality
- Avoid Comparison
- Sandwich Generation

5

Care Choices

- In-Home vs. Care Facility
- Connecting with Caregivers
- Relationships

6

End of Life Plans

- Plan Now then put away until the time comes
- Hospice Options

A Practical Guide to Dealing with a Dementia or Alzheimer's Diagnosis in the Family

by Tara Reed

Table of Contents

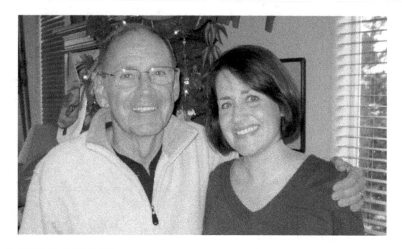

DEDICATION

This book is dedicated to my dad - George Reed. He is an amazing man, teacher, husband and father. The beginning and ending of his life is riddled with adversity; as a child, he lost his brother and both parents by the time he was 14. At 72, he was officially diagnosed with Alzheimer's. As I write this book, he is still with us but in a very different way.

I also dedicate this book to my family - my mom, Joan, my sister, Christine, my brother, Gary. To my son, Kyle and my husband, Craig. To Mike and Kelly. To Karen, Gillian, Bridger and Landon. To my friends, too numerous to name, who are always there for me when I need someone to listen and lean on. To our extended family and friends. Without everyone's love and support, this journey would be even harder - my continued gratitude to each and every one of you.

INTRODUCTION

Welcome to *What to Do Between the Tears: A Practical Guide to Dealing with a Dementia or Alzheimer's Diagnosis in the Family*. I'm sorry you are reading this. I assume it is because you, too, are looking for answers, guidance and advice about how to navigate the time ahead. I want to begin by telling you a little bit about myself and why I'm writing this book.

There are so many ways to describe who we are - labels that we put on ourselves and others, roles that we play, hats that we wear. "My name is Tara Reed and my dad has Alzheimer's." is one way to describe me. Here is more about who I am, who I am not and what my intentions are with this book.

I am not...

- an attorney, accountant or licensed psychiatrist.
- a neurologist or medical professional of any sort.

This means that the information I share is not legal or medical advice and should not be relied on as such. It is my understanding of how things work and should be used as a guide to help you decide what you may want to investigate for your specific situation. Please seek out expert advice before making big decisions; it will be worth the money and peace of mind in the end.

I am...

- a daughter of dementia and Alzheimer's - my father was officially diagnosed in 2012 but we began figuring things out years before. "We" being my family - my mother, sister, brother and me.
- an artist and a writer.
- a wife and mother.
- an optimistic realist - a silver lining specialist.
- organized. I have a talent for looking at the big picture and putting it into smaller, more manageable pieces so I and others can move forward.
- an action taker and when necessary, a swift, massive action taker.

I believe...

- we are meant to be happy and that we can find a lesson or silver lining in any adversity.
- we can decide if adversity will make us stronger or make us victims.
- we always have a choice - about what to do and what to focus on. Sometimes we think there is only one choice, but that is because the consequences of any other choice are unacceptable to us. There is ALWAYS more than one choice.

My intention is...

- to create a usable guide to help others navigate their way through what is to come when a family member or friend is diagnosed with dementia or Alzheimer's.
- to give you a resource to turn to when you don't know what to do.
- to empower you with knowledge and help you see the difference between what you can and can't control.
- to help you find peace whenever possible.
- to share personal stories to illustrate my journey and help you see that you are not alone as things happen in your life.

Now that you know a little bit more about who I am let's dive in!

– Tara Reed

P.S. I live in the United States so most of the resources noted in this book are U.S. based. If you live in another part of the world, head to the internet and find resources that are available in your country!

P.P.S. I have more resources on my website at
www.PivotToHappy.com/alz/

"No man is an island, entire of itself."
- John Donne

Part 1:
Diagnosis

"A journey of a thousand miles,
begins with a single step."
– Confucius

Unless dementia comes on suddenly, as a result of an accident or surgery, a diagnosis usually comes long after you suspect something is wrong.

My dad was diagnosed in 2012 and has been in a memory care home since May of 2013. Looking back, we can see the forgetfulness and personality changes were emerging for at least 10 years.

It's a tricky business – because most people are aging as the signs appear, and not all forgetfulness is dementia or Alzheimer's. You wonder, "Is he just getting old? Is he just turning into a grumpy old man or is something else at work here?"

It started off with little things. Forgetfulness... what was that person's name? Where did I put the keys? He looked to my mom to fill in the gaps in stories of their life. Then it grew – my dad went from being a conversationalist to a deliverer of monologues about his life. He would tell us things that he had done, accomplished and seen as if we didn't know – or didn't care. It was a rough few years trying to patiently listen to the same stories over and over again... sometimes he could go on for hours!

My dad has a degree in Physics and a doctorate in Science Education. He taught Astronomy at West Chester University for over 30 years. He wrote a weekly newspaper article (that was required reading in my high school Physics class!) about naked eye astronomy. Each week he would tell you what to look for in the night sky. It has now been three years since he has known night from day.

I vividly remember standing outside of an adult day care, where he thought he was a volunteer, at 9:30 pm, in the Oregon rain, trying to explain why I thought it was night. (It was dark!) At 8:50 PM he insisted it was time to go to work and told my mom he would walk if she wouldn't take him. As he left the house she decided to drive him to show him the place was closed. When he got out of the car and wasn't swayed by the locked doors and lack of lights, she called me in a panic. My husband and I headed there to see what we could do.

I tried to use terms he might relate to, "Remember dad, the earth turns on its axis and when we are away from the sun it's dark, it is night. We sleep at night, it's not when you come here and work."

"Who makes up these rules?" he asked, extremely agitated and frustrated.

"Don't you believe me?" I replied.

Everyday things get confusing to someone with dementia...

He thought about that and said, "I don't think you would lie to me but it doesn't make sense."

We finally got him to agree to go home after my brother called the Alzheimer's Association hotline for help. They told my brother to have someone call my dad, say they were a person he knew that worked at the facility, and explain that they had an emergency and had to close. My sister-in-law's boss called my phone, told my dad there was a water main break and that they would call him when it was time to come back.

My dad accepted this with no problem. This was our first lesson in "jumping into their reality". There comes a point where what is real to them is the only thing that matters, so you jump in with them until their reality shifts again.

It's hard to believe that was less than three years ago. Now he is very withdrawn, speaks softly if he speaks at all. I'm surprised and delighted if he comes up with a 3-4 word sentence that makes sense.

**Because of my father's Alzheimer's,
my perspective on life has changed.**

While I know that we all have an expiration date, I never expected my dad's final years to be like this or for this to be my family's experience. I've learned, even more so than before, to be present in the day I'm given. I don't take for granted having another 30-40 years. Carpe Diem has a whole new meaning!

Dementia and Alzheimer's - Defined

Dictionary.com defines dementia as severe impairment or loss of intellectual capacity and personality integration, due to the loss of or damage to neurons in the brain.

Loss or damage to the brain are key components to dementia. Sometimes symptoms that seem like dementia may be due to vitamin deficiencies or thyroid issues so most doctors will rule those out first.

My dad was given vitamin B to see if his symptoms changed, they didn't. Later an MRI showed that he had vascular dementia, which is when blood flow stops to areas of the brain - often as a result of strokes. At first we were told he didn't have Alzheimer's - we later found out he has both.

Dementia is a broad term for a decline in mental ability that is severe enough to interfere with daily life. Memory loss is a common example. Alzheimer's is the most common type of dementia and accounts for 60-80% of dementia according to the Alzheimer's Association.
(http://www.alz.org/what-is-dementia.asp)

The term dementia is sort of like the word virus - it is a general term, like an umbrella that covers many specific issues. There are many types of viruses and many causes of dementia. In this book I will talk about dementia in general and more specifically Alzheimer's. We have had friends who were told their loved ones had different types of dementia, only to find out after they passed away and had a brain autopsy, that the diagnosis was incorrect and they did indeed have Alzheimer's.

Alzheimer's is caused by plaques and tangles in the brain; physical compounds and fibers that build up in the brain and cause damage, as opposed to damage from lack of blood to the area. (Vascular dementia.)   Plaques are deposits of a protein fragment called beta-amyloid that builds up in the spaces between nerve cells, eventually blocking communication between those cells. Tangles are twisted fibers of another protein called tau that build up inside cells and also negatively impact the cellular function in the brain. When the brain starts to have problems, the rest of the body follows.

Beta-amyloid and tau fibers can be detected with a spinal tap, and was in my father's case, although I believe it's unusual to have this done. Final confirmation of an Alzheimer's diagnosis is usually done by an autopsy of the brain once the person is deceased.

There are many unknowns when it comes to how people get Alzheimer's and the high levels of plaques and tangles associated with it (most people have some as they age but not enough to impair the ability to function). There is a lot of research being done to better understand dementia and Alzheimer's and many clinical trials to find a way to slow the symptoms and progress. At this point, there is no cure for this progressive disease.

(Learn more: www.alz.org/alzheimers_disease_what_is_ alzheimers.asp#tangles)

Patient Reactions to a Diagnosis

It's not an easy cure because our brains are so complex. They are the compilation of a lifetime of connections, health, thoughts and more. Each person's experience affects how their brain is wired and so each experience of decline will be unique as well.

Diagnosing dementia isn't cut and dry either; there isn't a blood test that gives a yes or no answer. Each person's mental capacity is different and how they are impacted varies. How they perform on cognitive tests is different at their prime and during their decline. My dad had an amazing memory and was an excellent test taker. So the cognitive tests they give at the doctor's office weren't hard for him. I was there during one of these tests and I think he did better than I would have done - even though earlier in the day he forgot my brother's name 3 times.

Many become unsure of themselves or do their best to cover - they inherently know that something is wrong but try not to let on.

Everyone reacts differently to a diagnosis and many patients have lost too much cognitive ability to understand what it means. From my experience talking to other families, it seems like less than half the people with dementia ever understand that anything is wrong with them. I look at it as a blessing and as a curse. It's a blessing because understanding that you have an incurable disease would be hard to swallow.

It's a curse because it makes things harder on the family. Believing they are fine, they don't understand why they can't be as independent as they were before. They can be very frustrated, which often triggers resentment and anger. They think they are fine yet people are telling them what they can and can't do.

If they do understand, they can be involved in planning for care and will likely need different kinds of support to come to terms with the disease. I have seen people accept it with graceful resignation and others sink into depression.

My dad never understood or acknowledged that he had a problem. I vividly remember sitting in the neurologist's office with him and my mother as the neurologist delivered the diagnosis. We decided to ask the neurologist to tell him he had Alzheimer's, knowing he would argue with us but hoping he would accept it from a doctor.

He was sitting on the table, wearing a button down shirt under a white fleece with a name tag on his chest from a job he had left decades ago. He looked at the doctor and listened to her calmly. My mom and I were on chairs facing him, our backs to the wall, the door to my left, my mom to my right. We were both nervous, knots in our stomach, unsure of how he would react.

The doctor told him she had his test results and that not only did he have vascular dementia, but the spinal tap she had done 2 weeks earlier revealed that he had Alzheimer's as well.

He just looked at her and without emotion said, "No I don't."

My mom and I exchanged panicked glances. My mom leaned forward and said, "George, do you know what that means? Do you understand what Alzheimer's is?"

Then my dad got angry. "I *DO NOT* have that. I am *FINE.*" He looked at the doctor then turned and pointed an accusatory finger at my mom and said, "*SHE* is the problem! The next thing she is going to do is find a doctor who says I have cancer and I don't have that either!"

We sat there stunned. Of all the scenarios we had come up with, this wasn't one of them. Looking back I feel as if it was probably good that he never understood what was happening. Since there is no cure, I think he has been happier and more content not knowing what was in his future.

It wasn't easier for my mom, his wife of 50 years, being attacked and accused of wanting him to be sick. Part of her knew it was the disease talking but another part was hurt to the core.

One of the silver linings I have found in this devastating disease is that the person doesn't suffer, at least not in a physical sense. There is confusion and sometimes fear, but there is not usually physical pain. It's the rest of the family and friends that go through the gamut of emotion and grieve the loss of someone who is still here.

There is a reason it's often called *"The Long Goodbye"*.

Telling Friends and Family

Deciding when and how to tell friends and family can be yet another stressful piece of the puzzle. The more people that know what is going on the less you can stay in denial... but it can also mean more help and support as well.

It is important to tell those close to you and your loved one what is happening before posting anything on social media. Also consider the awareness and feelings of the person diagnosed before posting on social media as well. My mom asked me to keep things very quiet for a full year, afraid that my dad would find out or it would somehow negatively impact him in his past professional community. I have to admit that I didn't completely agree with her but did respect her wishes. When it was the one year anniversary of his official diagnosis and he had been in a memory care home for 4 months, I did push to be able to talk about what was going on. I felt it would not only help me to be able to share but also help others that I was connected to online who were going through similar struggles.

Once we knew there was a definite problem, we began to make a list of people that we felt should get a call from one of us to let them know. This included family members and some close friends. Knowing that these would be hard conversations, we often chose a point person for different branches of the family and asked them to let others know. Over time we then connected with more people, some reaching out to us to offer help or sympathy, others we reached out to when we felt strong enough.

I was the one to make a lot of the calls, first because it gave me some sense of "doing something" and not feeling so helpless and because I thought (and my family agreed) that I would get through the conversations with fewer tears.

My dad never knew we made these calls and would have been angry if we told him since he never believed there was a problem. I explained that to the friends and family I talked with and asked them to respect that and not question my dad directly. Our entire extended family was in Pennsylvania where my parents grew up and raised us. Since my brother, my parents and I had all moved west, at different times and for different reasons in the mid-90's, we had little in-person contact. Letting them know what was happening gave many relatives a chance to reach out and talk with my dad while he was still relatively well, without saying they knew what was going on. Had we waited too long, they wouldn't have been able to reconnect before things got really bad.

We kept the list of names and numbers, knowing that at some point in the future, a different type of call and notification would need to be made...

Things to consider...

- Consider the feelings and awareness of the person with dementia or Alzheimer's. Let friends and family know what is going on but also let them know whether the person is aware or not. Give them guidance about what to say if they decide to call or visit.
- Be sure close friends and family know what is happening before you say anything on social media. You may never choose to talk about it on social media, but you certainly don't want people close to your loved one to find out online.
- Think about who needs a personal call and who might be ok learning from another relative.
- Keep your list of names and numbers so it will be easy to find later.
- Some people will ask if there is anything they can do. Consider what help you might need so you are ready if the question arises. Don't be too proud to ask for help. This could be a long journey, so accept all the help you need!

Learning More About What is to Come...

Once there is an official diagnosis you will want to learn what to expect and what you can do, if anything. You, your family and friends will have many emotional responses as well. Grief and fear are common but come in a variety of ways.

As the biological child of someone with Alzheimer's, you might worry about the genetic factors involved and whether you are now more likely to develop Alzheimer's as well.

My dad has three biological children: me, my older sister and my younger brother. We all reacted differently to his diagnosis. My sister believes the whole illness is a crapshoot. Some people will get it, others won't, there isn't much we can do about it, so live your life and don't stress out.

I went on a 2 year journey looking for scientific indicators (short of the genetic test that is supposed to show a predisposition because if I can't do anything about it, I don't want that threat hanging over my head). I was looking for things I could control. Diet. Exercise. How well my body does or does not get rid of toxins. In my mind, I'm the most likely of the three of us to get Alzheimer's if there is a genetic component because I'm the most chemically like my dad. We both have B- blood which is very rare. Less than 2% of the world's population has B- blood (source: http://www.oneblood. org/target-your-type/b-negative.stml) We tend to have low blood pressure and also get shocked by door handles, even in the summer.

When my dad was diagnosed, my brother "just knew" he would one day get it too. I'm not sure why, and his reaction really surprised me. Maybe it's because he's the son and it's our dad who is affected. Hopefully he is wrong. Hopefully I am too!

Experts divide Alzheimer's into two groups: early-onset (when it occurs between the ages of 30 and 60) and late-onset (when it occurs in the mid-60s and beyond.)

According to the National Institute for Aging, early-onset Alzheimer's disease represents less than 5 percent of all people with Alzheimer's. Most cases of early-onset ARE due to genetic mutations, and a child whose biological mother or father carries a genetic mutation for early-onset Alzheimer's has a 50/50 chance of inheriting that mutation. If the mutation is in fact inherited, the child has a very strong probability of developing early-onset Alzheimer's.

There is no definitive link between specific genes and late-onset Alzheimer's and most believe it is a combination of genetics, environmental and lifestyle factors. (Or as my sister says, a crapshoot.)

(source: www.nia.nih.gov/alzheimers/publication/alzheimers-disease-genetics-fact-sheet)

Shortly after my dad was diagnosed with vascular dementia and before the Alzheimer's diagnosis, my brother and I went to an informational meeting at OHSU (Oregon Health & Science University) in Portland, Oregon to learn more. The Layton Aging & Alzheimer's Disease Center (at OHSU) is one of

27 National Institutes for Health and Alzheimer's disease Centers in the United States and the only one of its kind in Oregon. We felt fortunate to have this resource in our own backyard. They are doing a lot of research at OHSU and the talk was given by one of the lead doctors.

The doctor explained the difference between vascular dementia and Alzheimer's and then talked about lifestyle changes people could make to decrease their risks. Things like maintaining a healthy weight, eating right, exercising and keeping your blood pressure under control. Check, check, check - our dad had done all these things.

We felt very young in a room full of gray hair with the seniors hanging onto the doctor's every word. When it came time for Q&A, several hands shot up.

"What about doing crossword puzzles and Sudoku to keep the mind working?" a woman asked. Many nodded their heads and sat up in anticipation of the answer. It seemed a valid question since so many advise keeping your brain active as a way to stave off dementia... we knew it wasn't going to be a "miracle fix" since our dad used his brain extensively and was still affected. He read, he wrote, he studied - I can't remember many hours in a day when my dad wasn't actively engaged.

The doctor smiled and replied, "It is hard to scientifically measure the effect of crossword puzzles and Sudoku. We know many people are doing these activities in the hopes of preventing dementia. It is good to keep your brain active, but it's hard to know if it will make a difference. We may just have a new generation of dementia and Alzheimer's patients who are good at crossword puzzles and Sudoku." This wasn't the answer people were looking for.

(Some research suggests Sudoku can help: www.robwinningham.com/blog/2014/02/08/crossword-puzzles-are-not-as-good-as-sudoku-puzzles-for-exercising-the-brain/)

> "If you've met one person with Alzheimer's, you've met one person with Alzheimer's. Each will have a different path."

The doctor also said something that has stayed with me and that I've shared with many people: "If you've met one person with Alzheimer's, you've met one person with Alzheimer's." He explained that each person's experience and path is different, so learning every detail about the decline of your neighbor's grandmother won't necessarily prepare you to deal with your own grandmother's decline. If a loved one gets a dementia and possible Alzheimer's diagnosis, learn what you can but know that your experience will be unique.

My best advice when it comes to learning about what is to come is to trust your gut. You will know how much you want to learn and when you have had enough. Also remember that people can put anything on the internet - so if something seems off, investigate further. Talk to your doctors about it.

Also remember that we all come to things, including dementia and Alzheimer's, with our own lens and filter. Doctors, for example, are trained to look for solutions to sustain life as long as possible. Once a person goes on hospice, the focus shifts to comfort measures and not alleviating symptoms. You will encounter a wide range of views about what you should do, how you should feel and who you should talk to. Do what makes the most sense to YOU and your family.

Some resources to learn more about what is happening in the brain:

- **Alzheimer's Association** - I'll refer to them a lot as they have an amazing resource of knowledge! www.alz.org
- **What is dementia?** www.alz.org/what-is-dementia.asp
- **What is Alzheimer's?** www.alz.org/alzheimers_disease_what_is_alzheimers.asp
- **10 Early Signs and Symptoms of Alzheimer's** www.alz.org/alzheimers_disease_10_signs_of_alzheimers.asp
- **Stages of Alzheimer's** www.alz.org/alzheimers_disease_stages_of_alzheimers.asp
- **Inside the Brain: An Interactive Tour** www.alz.org/alzheimers_disease_4719.asp
- **National Institute on Aging** www.nia.nih.gov
- **About Alzheimer's Disease:** www.nia.nih.gov/alzheimers/topics/alzheimers-basics

---

Pharmaceuticals, Clinical Trials and Nutrition...

The decision to try medication or look into clinical trials is a very personal one. I'm going to share my understanding and some stories I've heard and then you can decide what you want to look into and try. Remember that I'm not a doctor; I'm sharing what I've learned through my own reading and research.

Right now there is no cure for Alzheimer's. There is a lot of scientific research being done in the hope of finding a cure. For now, there are drug and non-drug treatments that may help with both cognitive and behavioral symptoms.

Pharmaceuticals

Let's start with drugs - government approved pharmaceuticals your doctor may recommend. The goal of medication is to see if they lessen the symptoms or slow down the progress of the disease. Nothing can reverse or cure the dementia or Alzheimer's.

The U.S. Food and Drug Administration (FDA) has approved two types of medications — cholinesterase inhibitors (Aricept, Exelon, Razadyne) and memantine (Namenda) — to treat the cognitive symptoms (memory loss, confusion, and problems with thinking and reasoning) of Alzheimer's disease. It is my understanding that they cannot repair the damage that has been done in the brain, but they may slow down the progression of the disease or stabilize symptoms. Some doctors prescribe one type, but others prescribe both, to see what happens. As with any drug, there are a wide variety of potential side effects. Be sure to ask questions, do your research and make sure the side effects are worth the potential benefit.

It is very tempting to try anything and to trust your doctors implicitly. Be sure to find a doctor or team of doctors that you trust but also know that you can choose to use medications or not. I have heard of people who didn't realize they had a choice and that they could say "no thank you" to a doctor's recommendation.

Here are things to consider when deciding whether to try medications:

- Where is your loved one NOW in the disease? Are they in a place (behavior, memory, and contentedness) that they and you would want to stay if the medication worked and slowed down the progress?
- How do they usually react to medication? Do they do well or do they often have a lot of side effects?
- Weigh the pros and cons of slowing down symptoms - will it maintain and/or extend quality of life or just quantity?
- What is your goal?

We tried medication for my dad briefly. It didn't help his anxiety and anger but did have some very unfortunate stomach related side effects. In the end we chose to stop the medication since there were no significant benefits. There were people who judged us for the decision, but in our hearts we knew it was what my dad would have wanted when he was healthy and what was best for our family.

I know of other people who have tried medications with great results. Their loved one was content and became stabilized in a good place with few side effects.

The choice to try and use medications is a decision that each family needs to make. We also need to respect the choices made by others, even if they differ from our opinion of what should be done. When friends approach me, worried that their friend or parent may be going down the road to dementia, my advice is this: "If you think you want to try medication to slow it down, try it sooner rather than later. It works better in the early stages, but most people I have met don't realize what is happening until a later stage when the medications seem less effective or people are stalled in confusion or anger."

Make your own choice. Follow your heart. Don't be pressured in either direction and don't feel obliged to share your decisions with the world if you don't want to.

In addition to the drugs mentioned above to help stabilize or delay symptoms from brain deterioration, your loved one may need medication for other issues that often come with an Alzheimer's or dementia diagnosis.

Commonly treated symptoms include:

- depression
- sleeplessness or disruptive sleep cycles
- behavior problems like agitation, aggression, obsessive-compulsive behavior, paranoia, etc.

Where to learn more:

- www.alz.org/alzheimers_disease_standard_prescriptions.asp
- Do searches on each specific drug to see potential side effects.
- Talk with others to see what their experience has been but know that every person will react and respond differently.

Clinical Trials

Clinical trials are done before the FDA approves a drug into the marketplace and before any claims can be made about what a drug can prevent or cure. The final stages of FDA approval involves carefully monitored and documented clinical trials with volunteers. Without clinical trials, advances in medical science can't be made.

That said, this too is a very personal decision. Talk to your doctor to see if they know of any studies being done in your area or look into the Alzheimer's Association TrialMatch.

TrialMatch is a free clinical studies matching service that connects individuals with Alzheimer's, caregivers, healthy volunteers and physicians with current studies. They continuously update the database of Alzheimer's clinical trials and it currently includes more than 225 promising clinical studies being conducted at nearly 700 trial sites across the country.

Learn more: www.alz.org/research/clinical_trials/find_clinical_trials_trialmatch.asp

Nutrition

Good nutrition is important for everyone - from birth to death - to help support the body to function properly. As we age, each person may be faced with different body systems not working optimally, from high cholesterol to blood pressure issues to diabetes, weight gain and more. Genetics contribute to some and others are more related to environmental exposures, lifestyle choices and nutrition.

There are many theories and claims about supplements (sometimes called Nutraceuticals to sound more scientific) or nutrition regimes to help prevent, stop or halt dementia and Alzheimer's. Since they are not regulated by the FDA, everything you read may not be fact, or not enough fact that it would pass the stringent approval requirements.

There are people passionately for and against the FDA legislations and enforcement. It's up to you to decide which side of the debate you fall on, but it is good to understand why the rules are in place. They are designed to protect the average consumer from the proverbial snake oil salesman.

When people learn that you have a family member with dementia or Alzheimer's - they will send you every article or quick fix they see. They do it because they want to ease your pain and help you find a solution. It is then up to you to do your research and decide if it is something you want to try.

One nutrient you will certainly read and hear about when you begin doing your research is coconut oil. There is a lot of talk about coconut oil being a miracle cure for Alzheimer's. I've seen a video about a man who, after eating it on his toast every morning, had a miraculous reversal of symptoms. This gave a lot of hope to people - but this is the only case I've heard of with this type of result. After we heard about it, we tried giving my dad coconut oil but saw no change or improvement. There was no harm in trying, but we were disappointed that we didn't have the same results as the man in the video. I now use coconut oil regularly because of the health benefits I learned about when doing research for my dad and I hope this lifestyle change keeps me healthier than I may have been.

Another common miracle cure you will read about is turmeric. There are a multitude of blog posts and articles that say, "consuming turmeric will prevent and cure Alzheimer's." The words "prevent" and "cure" put these bloggers or companies at risk of having the FDA come after them unless they have the research to prove it.

Claims like that are often generalizations based on ongoing research and medical papers - so not always a hoax, but not yet scientifically proven.

Here is an article I found on the National Institute for Health's website.

"Curcumin (Turmeric), an ancient Indian herb used in curry powder, has been extensively studied in modern medicine and Indian systems of medicine for the treatment of various medical conditions, including cystic fibrosis, hemorrhoids, gastric ulcer, colon cancer, breast cancer, atherosclerosis, liver diseases and arthritis. It has been used in various types of treatments for dementia and traumatic brain injury. Curcumin also has a potential role in the prevention and treatment of Alzheimer's disease. Curcumin as an antioxidant, anti-inflammatory and lipophilic action improves the cognitive functions in patients with Alzheimer's disease. A growing body of evidence indicates that oxidative stress, free radicals, beta amyloid, cerebral deregulation caused by bio-metal toxicity and abnormal inflammatory reactions contribute to the key event in Alzheimer's disease pathology. Due to various effects of curcumin, such as decreased Beta-amyloid plaques, delayed degradation of neurons, metal-chelation, anti-inflammatory, antioxidant and decreased microglia formation, the overall memory in patients with Alzheimer's disease has improved. This paper reviews the various mechanisms of actions of curcumin in Alzheimer's disease and pathology.

The process through which Alzheimer's disease degrades the nerve cells is believed to involve certain properties: inflammation, oxidative damage and most notably, the formation of beta-amyloid plaques, metal toxicity."

(source: www.ncbi.nlm.nih.gov/pmc/articles/PMC2781139/)

To summarize, researchers are looking at potential causes of Alzheimer's (inflammation, metal toxicity, plaques, etc.) and then natural compounds that help combat the causes. In this case, they are studying the effect of Curcumin - an element of the spice Turmeric - on inflammation, metal toxicity and plaques.

It's a lot easier to say "Turmeric will prevent Alzheimer's" and get the average reader's attention than to go into the science of it.

Will Turmeric alone prevent or cure Alzheimer's? The jury is out. The incidence of the disease in India, where Turmeric is a more common ingredient in their diet, is less than in the US. Is it the only variable? Probably not.

I want there to be a quick fix to all of this. I want to put coconut oil on my toast and know that I will be fine. I wish the Turmeric we put in my dad's smoothies had stopped his decline and reversed the effects. (Yes, we tried it! Our feeling was "Why not? It won't hurt and there is a slim chance it will help.") But for now, I don't see quick fixes working.

Do your research. If there are potential health benefits and few risks or negative side effects, by all means, try whatever it is. Use them yourself; see if they help your loved one. But watch for side effects and beware of the emotional roller coaster you could jump on if you get your hopes up only to find there is no notable change.

Eat real food with the nutrients your body needs to function at its best. Feed your loved one well too. Reduce your exposure to toxins and chemicals that could cause long-term harm. Manage stress in your life. Look at lifestyle elements and see where you can improve. But live and enjoy your life too. Balance is key.

How do People with Alzheimer's Die?

One of the big questions we had when my dad was first diagnosed was "How do people with Alzheimer's actually die?" Many death certificates don't put Alzheimer's or dementia as a cause of death - even though it is said to be the 6th leading cause of death in the US.

(Source & other statistics:
www.alz.org/facts/overview.asp#mortality)

My understanding is that Alzheimer's usually contributes to another issue that becomes the final cause of death. The brain deteriorates and the body is weakened. It is often a heart attack, stroke or infection that ends the person's life. Surgery, due to a fall or injury, also begins the spiral to the end of life for many.

Changing Roles and Relationships

When a loved one is diagnosed with dementia or Alzheimer's, the roles and relationships can feel like they change overnight. The diagnosis is often the wakeup call where you can no longer wish that the behavior is just a phase and that it will get better - you know it will only get worse. You are no longer just a husband or wife, a daughter or son, a friend... you are now a caregiver or support person as well.

Remember that changing roles in life is natural. Some roles you are excited to take on, like becoming an adult and going out on your own. People are excited to get married and move from being a girlfriend or boyfriend to a wife or husband. When you have your first child you become a parent - it's a huge change in your role and responsibility!

Unfortunately few people are excited to step into the role of caregiver for a spouse or parent. But stepping up to the challenge is vital for the health and well-being of everyone involved, especially your loved one.

Some people are born caregivers and others find it to be extremely hard. If caregiving is a strength and a calling, you will likely choose to keep your loved one at home longer than someone who struggles to adapt. It is important to be honest and figure out where your strengths are and get help where you need it. Natural caregivers are no better than those who have a harder time adapting to a less independent partner; it just is or isn't who you are. Don't judge yourself or others, just find a way to get the job done.

To use my family as an example, my mother is the obvious caregiver for my dad. They are married and had lived together for 48 years when an MRI confirmed vascular dementia. When we had scientific proof that there was a problem that wasn't going to get better, we began to strongly suggest my parents move to Portland, Oregon. They had been living in Nevada for almost 20 years but had no family there. My sister lived in Pennsylvania, where my family is originally from, and both my brother and I now live in Portland. We could see the writing on the wall - our mom and dad, would need more than phone support and we would all feel better if we could be in closer proximity for what was to come.

My mom resisted, regularly saying she didn't want to move "because she didn't want it to affect our lives." It was going to affect our lives either way. It was our dad! She was trying to protect us from what she had been dealing with for years. My dad had been resistant to moving as well, but I can't remember why.

I do remember convincing him to consider moving while in a parking lot near my house. My parents were in town a few weeks before my wedding, helping go over some last minute decisions and visiting my brother's twins who were 1 and growing fast!

"Dad, I think you should move to Portland!"

"Why? Your mom and I like Nevada."

"Because we miss you. I'm going to be staying here and Gary, his wife and kids (3 cute little kids) are here. You could see your grandkids more and we could see each other more. It would be great!"

Before he could form an objection I continued, "If you could have your ideal house, what would it have in it?" We began to talk about his dream office where he could store all his books and do his writing. We discussed how he loves a view of the mountains and would like to be close to downtown. I pointed out how awesome it would be for them to be able to see family without a twelve hour drive from Reno.

My mom just looked at me dumbfounded; amazed that I had him thinking about it and shrugged when I asked if I could call my realtor. He was available the next day and we went and looked at some different areas. My parents went back to Nevada and put their house on the market.

When they returned in the beginning of August for my wedding, they had an offer on their house. My sister was in Portland for the wedding too so the family hunt for the perfect home for our parents began. We wanted a master bedroom on the main floor, trying to plan ahead in case stairs became an issue. We found an amazing house only 4 miles from my home. They put in an offer and moved a month later.

Getting most of the family in the same city was a big first step in dealing with what was to come. The move was just in time too. We didn't realize how bad things were until the move was taking place. My dad had been coping and hiding just how bad he was, but the stress of packing and moving made a lot more come to light.

Looking back, they should have moved a few years earlier. But my parents have always been incredibly independent and since we all lived so far apart, we didn't fully grasp how bad things were and how much stress our mom was under.

While we hadn't had any formal discussions, it was understood that my mom would be the main caregiver and I would be the backup. I lived close to their new house, worked from home and my son left for college a week before my parents move. My brother had small children, was a firefighter who worked 24 hour shifts near my parent's new house but lived over an hour away so his time was less flexible. My sister was 3,000 miles away. Her role would be to support everyone by phone and come out when she could.

Notes, Things to Research, Memories and More...

Part 2:
Planning for the Present and the Future

"If you fail to plan, you are planning to fail."
– Benjamin Franklin

As emotional as this time can be, it's a good idea to get a snapshot of where the person, couple or family are from a financial, legal and emotional standpoint. Look at where your loved one is as far as behavior, support and safety considerations and the skills and needs of the family who are now wearing the additional hats of caregiver or supporter. Finally look at medical options and wishes.

As I mentioned in the introduction, I feel better when I feel as if I'm in control and able to take action, so this was where my strengths come to light. Of course there is a lot we can't control with dementia but there are things we can control or manage.

The legal aspects of dementia, mental competency and end of life decisions should also be addressed as soon as possible - hopefully while the person is still legally able to make decisions and sign binding legal documents.

If you don't like to look at or deal with unpleasant realities, I get it. But it's time to take a deep breath and get it done. If you focus and work quickly, you can get these less than fun things sorted out and then go back to focusing on the positive and taking care of yourself and your loved one. If you don't take the time to assess what you have in place and make adjustments to legal, financial and medical matters now, you may find your state involved more than you would like and taking up time and valuable resources.

Many people will find they have nothing in place, if that is your case, the time is now. Also consider planning for your own future while you are thinking about these topics.

What we did and what I highly recommend you do is to gather as much data as possible. I have some lists to get you started in the following sections. Then find an elder law attorney in your state so you can fully understand your options. We spoke with two different attorneys to get two opinions and found one we really felt comfortable with; it was money well spent for the peace of mind and knowledge we gained.

FINANCIAL

Money is a huge concern when you are faced with the care of someone with dementia or Alzheimer's. Unless you have good long-term care insurance, it will take up a lot of financial resources. There are a lot of beliefs about how to protect your money or give it to your children so you don't have to pay for long-term care, but most are false. The rules and laws are confusing and you don't want to be on the wrong side of them.

Hopefully there has been money put away for a rainy day because as a cousin told my mom, "it's now raining."

What kind of financial assets does the person or couple have? Get as many details as possible, bank names, account numbers, contact people, balances, etc.

- Income (job, disability, rental property, etc.)
- Checking Account(s)
- Savings Account(s)
- Investment Account(s)
- Mutual funds
- Stocks
- Bonds
- Other
- Social Security
- Pension
- Retirement Fund
- Health Savings Account(s)
- Real Estate - value of any property owned and any associated debt (mortgages, etc.)
- Other Property - value of cars, boats, etc.
- Life Insurance - value / beneficiary(ies)
- Rights or Interest in Trusts, Estates or Inheritances
- Interest in a Business / Businesses
- Other assets or interests that have a monetary value

You should also review the beneficiaries of any of these accounts and talk to the elder law attorney about whether any of those should be adjusted.

Does your loved one have unlimited access to money, credit cards and computers? If they have traditionally been the person in charge of paying bills and making financial decisions, the time is now to move the responsibility to someone else.

I've heard many stories about people being duped into giving money to email and internet scams, or buying boats or cars or other expensive items because they still had access to money but didn't know better. You don't put a 6 year old in charge of your investments or checking account so don't leave someone with dementia in charge either. It's never too early to safeguard your assets; you will need them for the times ahead.

While you need to protect your money, you also need to protect the dignity of your loved one and not create extreme stress in your home. What my mom did was slowly remove credit cards from my dad's wallet. She also left him with no more than $10 in cash. At this point, he wasn't driving so he wasn't ever out and in need of money without her. He still wanted to have money and if he wandered and got lost, he could buy food or get a cab. He had a basic cell phone with our numbers as the favorites so someone could look at his phone and call us. He also wore a medic alert bracelet.

LEGAL DOCUMENTS

While it is important for everyone to have plans in place in case of an emergency, it is especially important when someone becomes terminally ill or dementia sets in. The following are some important legal documents you should have in place and reviewed by an elder law attorney to make sure you and your family will be able to make decisions for your loved one and have access to assets and money needed for their care.

Samples of basic health planning documents can usually be found on state government websites or at your doctor's office. Agencies on aging, state legal aid offices, and the State Bar Association may also provide legal advice or help.

Since most attorneys charge by the hour, take all financial and legal papers with you. Attorneys often send a list of important papers needed. Also think about the choices you will want to make so they can help you with the details.

- **A durable power of attorney for finances** - this legal form gives someone the power to make legal and financial decisions on behalf of the person with Alzheimer's. If the person is married, the spouse may automatically have this power, as was the case with my parents. But what if something happens to my mom? We made sure there was a plan B and my siblings and I are now authorized to make financial decisions if her health should fail. Only give this type of power to someone who can be trusted to keep the person's best interest in mind and who won't abuse it. (Unfortunately children don't always pass that test - this is a time to be very careful and realistic as you are placing a lot of trust and control in the hands of others.)
- **A durable power of attorney for health care** - this appoints a person or several people

(called a trustee or trustees) the power to make healthcare decisions on behalf of the person with Alzheimer's. Be sure the people appointed understand the wishes of the person with Alzheimer's and will keep the person's preference in mind.

- **A living trust** - a living trust is a document that tells an appointed trustee how to distribute a person's property and money while they are still alive.
- **A living will** - this spells out the person's wishes for end-of-life health care. This will include choices about feeding tubes, transfusions, extreme measures, etc.
- **A do-not-resuscitate form** - this tells healthcare staff not to perform cardiopulmonary resuscitation (CPR) if a person's heart stops or if he or she stops breathing. If this is the person's wish, complete it and make sure it is on record with their doctor and present it to staff if the person is hospitalized or living in a care home. If they live at home, have it in an obvious place in case of an emergency. Emergency responders will often look on the refrigerator but if swift action needs to be taken, someone may need to tell them to stop, that there is a DNR.
- **A will** - a will tells how the person wants his or her property and money to be distributed after death. Many married people think they don't need a will because everything would automatically go to the surviving spouse. I believe that is true in most states, but I also think it's better to have it in writing just in case. There is no guarantee about who will pass away first,

and both could die at the same time in an accident. You may not want a person with dementia to be a sole beneficiary.

MEDICAL

There are two stages to medical considerations that you should consider and discuss as a family or support system: things that need to happen now and things that will become an issue later, as the disease progresses.

Let's start with things to consider and do now.

SAFETY

I like to begin with safety issues because these are vitally important and often things you aren't accustomed to thinking about when it concerns an adult. We automatically watch for safety with children because we know they may not have the knowledge or life experience to make good choices to be safe.

When the signs of dementia become more prevalent, you will need to look after your loved one as if they were a child again. Their ability to make decisions and stay safe will become impaired. These safety issues could be one of your biggest sources of conflict with the person and potentially with family members. I believe safety needs to trump all - and tough decisions need to be made to keep everyone safe.

Driving is a really hard thing to broach with any aging person and especially one with dementia. Our legal system makes it difficult for driving rights of the elderly to be revoked, and in my experience some doctors are hesitant to get involved. Our family had to make the decision, and it was very stressful and difficult. Figure out a way to get your loved one off the road before anyone is injured including innocent bystanders and other drivers.

Help them figure out how they will still be able to get around. What options are available? Is there public transportation for seniors in the area? Is there someone who can drive them places a few days a week? Can you hire someone to help? Use a cab? Get creative and help them keep some sense of independence while also keeping them and everyone else safe.

We were fortunate that Oregon requires any new resident to pass a knowledge exam to get a driver's license, even if they have a current license in another state. Not all states have that requirement and if the person isn't moving to a new state, it won't help you. My whole family wrote letters to the state saying that we didn't believe my dad should be given a license and told them why. This put a red flag on his name in the system. He didn't pass the test, but because of our written concerns, he was told he couldn't retake it until he had a note from his doctor. A doctor may be hesitant to take steps to have a person's license canceled, but they would not write a letter to the DMV stating a person should be allowed to drive if they are known to have dementia. We also "lost the keys" to his car (behind the washer). Interestingly enough my dad never asked to drive my mom's car and let her drive him around while he kept looking for the keys to his car.

One day, at breakfast, my dad agreed to sell his car. I had already figured out how and where we would do that, planner that I am! Because we had a plan in place, we were able to sell the car within a few hours. Thankfully my brother was a witness to the conversation because my mom and I were accused of both stealing his car and "selling it out from under him" multiple times. He was angry but he was also safe, as were the other drivers on the road.

My dad was obsessed with getting a new car for months and would point out cars that he liked in car lots when we would be driving. Eventually he forgot about it, but it did take a while. Just know that taking the keys and possibly selling the car may not be the end of the argument. It is worth staying strong on the matter to keep everyone safe.

Depending on the stage of your loved one's dementia, any or all of these things may be a factor that could affect their safety:

- **Impaired judgment** - they may forget how to use appliances, to turn off stove top burners, to not walk into the street when cars are coming, etc.

- **Changes in their senses** - as the brain becomes more affected, your loved one may have changes in vision, hearing, depth perception or sensitivity to temperature.

- **Disorientation** - they may be unable to recognize familiar things or get lost in places they have known all their lives. Some dementia patients can get lost for long periods of time, even overnight.

- **Physical changes** - balance often becomes an issue and your loved one could be at higher risk of falling and may eventually need a walker or wheelchair.

Be aware and on the lookout for signs that these or other things are becoming an issue. If balance becomes a problem, install safety bars in the bathroom and have a walker on hand just in case. Hold their hand on walks so they don't misjudge stairs or a sidewalk. Be there to assist without making them feel helpless. Pharmacies and doctors can be good resources for ideas about safety devices that can make life easier. You can also learn a lot by searching online for *Home Safety for People with Alzheimer's Disease*.

We were lucky that my dad never liked to cook anything that didn't require a microwave so the oven and stove top were never an issue. I've heard stories of people causing fires because they forgot they had turned a burner on under a pot and walked away. As long as your loved one is at home you need to constantly monitor their behavior so you know when new safety issues could occur.

Many people, like my dad, get what they call "Sundowners". It's as if their body clock gets reversed and they can be up and wandering throughout the night and sleeping during the day. When the person lives at home, it is taxing on a spouse or caregiver. The caregiver ends up not only stressed but also sleep deprived because their nights are spent listening for the person getting up.

Sundowners Syndrome: refers to behavioral changes that often occur in the late afternoon or evening.

We got a home security system that would ding whenever an exterior door was opened so we would know, day or night, if my dad tried to leave the house. This helped prevent him from going out alone and getting lost.

If your loved one wanders at all, consider getting ID jewelry for peace of mind. MedicAlert® + Alzheimer's Association Safe Return® is a 24-hour nationwide emergency response service for individuals with Alzheimer's or a related dementia who wander or have a medical emergency. They provide 24-hour assistance, no matter when or where the person is reported missing. You can get a bracelet or necklace that gives pertinent medical and contact information in case your loved one is found and can't give the information needed to get them home safely.

Learn more: www.alz.org/care/dementia-medic-alert-safe-return.asp#ixzz3nZBuM8VD

Some states, counties or cities also have programs for seniors who wander. Find out what the options are and decide what makes sense to you.

Cars can be a safety issue, even when your loved one isn't driving. My parents had planned to go to a museum my dad always liked, but on the way he thought he needed to be somewhere else. He got so angry that he jumped out of the car while my mom was coming to a stop at a red light on a 4 lane street. I got a frantic, tearful call from my mom as he walked up the road in the opposite direction. She finally convinced him to get back in the car and took him where he wanted to go. After that day she used the child safety locks so he couldn't open the door while she was driving.

Assess your home the way you would if a toddler was coming for a visit. Make your home as safe and comfortable as possible for your loved one so you don't have to hover and watch them 24/7. Reassess the safety measures you have in place every few months as their dementia and symptoms progress.

Places to start in regard to safety:

- Put sharp knives and other objects out of reach.
- Don't have firearms or weapons in the home unless they are disarmed and securely locked away.
- Keep medication out of reach.

- Consider safety knobs for stove top burners so they can't be turned on without your help.
- Remove tripping hazards.
- Install safety bars and equipment in bathrooms if mobility becomes an issue.
- Make sure you have working safety devices like fire alarms, fire extinguishers and carbon monoxide detectors.
- Have emergency numbers programmed into your phone and posted in your home.
- Remove or disable power tools that could cause harm.
- Post information in your home, usually in the kitchen, to let emergency responders know that your loved one has dementia so they will be better able to assess and assist them.

Assessing and Planning for your Current Support Needs

After you have taken care of immediate safety issues, it's time to look at where you are, what your strengths and skills are and what types of help you need. There are many ways to get help and many people who offer it.

Because of the cost of long term care, most people try to keep their loved one at home as long as possible. They say it takes a village to raise a child, but it often takes a village to move through the final years as well. Some villagers are volunteers, others will be paid help. It's time to figure out who you need in your village!

Let's assess, beyond safety issues, the abilities and needs of the person with dementia. This is also a good list to reassess every few months to make sure you make adjustments as needs change.

Communication Skills and Memory

- Can they verbalize their needs, hold conversations and communicate their feelings?
- Do they look confused when given too many options?
- Has their communication style changed - do they talk more, less or about different things than they used to?
- Do they lose words often or forget personal stories and memories?
- Do they misplace things regularly? Can they retrace their steps to find things?
- Are they often disoriented and unsure about their surroundings?

Personal Care

- Can they bathe or shower themselves?
- Is incontinence an issue?
- Can they brush their teeth and hair independently?
- Can they pick out their own clothes and dress themselves?
- Can they feed themselves? Can they prepare their own meals?
- Do they have trouble swallowing or have issues with hot or cold foods or drinks?

Motor Skills

- How is their balance? Have they fallen or do they trip more than usual?
- Can they walk well or do they shuffle their feet?
- Do they have trouble with fine motor skills - like picking up and manipulating small objects or has there been a change in their handwriting?
- Do their hands shake or do they have any other muscle tremors or twitches?
- Can they stand up, sit down and move well on their own?
- Are they more hesitant than they used to be? In general, on stairs, in unfamiliar places?

Interests and Energy Levels

- Do they sleep more or less than they used to?
- Have their sleep patterns changed? Are they napping in the day and up all night?
- Have their interests and activities changed substantially?
- Are they angrier than they used to be, more withdrawn, quiet or depressed?

Activities

- What do they like to do now? Create a list of things they enjoy doing so you have ways to engage with them or to divert their attention when necessary.

- Look for things they enjoy doing and make it part of a daily routine. Empower them to feel useful.
- Are there times of day when they are more engaged in activities than others? Watch for patterns to emerge and change over time.

If other things come to mind, be sure to make note of them. Every person will have different needs, likes and routines. These are some basic things to consider that will change as the disease progresses.

Now that you have taken some time to look at where they are still independent and where they need help, it's time to look at the support system that can be put in place.

First, who is the primary caregiver? It is usually the person living with the person with dementia. Is that person in good health? Do they have a support system in place and how are their stress levels? Are they able to provide the majority of care and do they have a way to get respite - no one can be an effective caregiver 24/7.

Many families have a family meeting - either formal or informal, to brainstorm and plan the near future. Are there siblings, children or extended family that can and are willing to help? Friends or neighbors who might lend a hand?

What skills does each person bring to the table? How much time are they willing to commit to help? Open and honest communication at the beginning and setting expectations can help avoid conflict down the road.

My family has managed to become a stronger, more cohesive unit through my dad's Alzheimer's, but I have seen and heard of many families that are torn apart.

I've heard of children who refuse to let one parent put another in a home but don't step up to help. It isn't fair to dictate what care will look like if you aren't ready to put time, energy and/or money into the solution.

We have always approached it from the standpoint of support, safety and dignity. What does dad need right now to be safe and content? What support does mom need to navigate the slow loss of her husband and figuring out what her life will look like now? What support do each of us need to deal with the stress and emotions of supporting both of our parents and dealing with the slow loss of our father?

We haven't always agreed on the right course of action, but we have always talked it out and listened to each other's perspectives. We have sought outside advice when we didn't have the knowledge or expertise to make a decision. Communication and respect are KEY.

Leave your super hero cape at the door. Everyone will have moments of strength and moments of emotional meltdown. The key to surviving and thriving is to know when you need to step away, when you can step in to carry the load, and when to ask for help.

After working through this section, you will have a better idea of the support your loved one diagnosed with dementia and/or Alzheimer's needs. You will also know which of those needs can be met by the primary caregiver and where they need support. It's time for more lists!

- What help does your loved one need when it comes to safety and personal care?
- Is there a trusted health care team in place?
- Is companionship and interaction available in addition to the primary caregiver?
- What would lighten the load of the primary caregiver?
- Housekeeping services?
- Food preparation?
- Respite care? (Respite care is basically getting a break - like hiring a babysitter or trading play dates when your kids are little so you can have some me-time. Caregivers need it too - we just call it respite care instead of babysitting.)
- What support does the primary caregiver have for their mental and physical health?
- Where can others fill in the gaps?
- Can someone offer to spend a few hours on a regular basis so the primary caregiver can leave and have a break?
- Can anyone provide overnight or weekend respite support?

Know your Support Options Beyond Friends and Family

Many people have no idea what services are available to help. There are many options and types of people to assist you. Here are a few:

- **Physicians** - Find a doctor you like and trust to help you understand your options and help care for your loved one.

- **Nutrition Programs** - Programs like Meals on Wheels or other organizations offer support with food and nutrition. Research what is available in your area. www.MealsOnWheelsAmerica.org

- **Home Care** refers to health care and supportive services to help homebound, sick or disabled persons continue living at home as independently as possible. Home Care falls under one of two categories: Home Health Care or Non-Medical Care.
  - **Home Health Care** provides medical services - help with medication, nursing services, physical therapy, etc.
  - **Non-Medical Care** includes help with household activities, personal care (bathing, dressing, eating), companionship, etc.
  - See if your insurance will cover the costs of home health care, they rarely cover non-medical care but it is worth asking!

- **Adult Day Care** is a great option to provide the primary caregiver some time off. It also offers social opportunities and activities for participants. Your loved one can enjoy peer support and receive health and social services in a safe, familiar environment at a fraction of the cost of living in a full time care home. It's often a great compromise between in or out of home living and care.

- **Support Groups** bring people together who are going through the same challenges you are. They meet regularly to share information and discuss practical solutions to common problems. Support groups can be a place to make friends and get support from your peers and professionals. They may be available from your state or local government, in hospitals, churches and more. You can also find support groups for specific diseases on association websites.

  The Alzheimer's Association has a page to help find support in your area: www.alz.org/apps/findus.asp

- **Advocacy Groups** - Many local and state agencies have some sort of advocacy program to help with issues concerning seniors. If you feel you need help understanding your options or advocating for your loved one, see what options are available to you.

- **Foster Care or Memory Care Facilities** - If it comes to a point where you can no longer care for your loved one in your home, there are different options.
  - **Foster Care Homes** - There are people who operate Foster Homes for seniors, where your loved one is in a home environment with a few other residents and cared for by licensed and trained caregivers. We toured a few when looking at options for my dad. Often it is a family business that may even have children in the home. One woman we met told us how the seniors would help her 10 year old son with his homework and ask about his day, acting as grandparent figures. It was good for their son and also made the residents feel important and useful.
  - **Memory Care Homes** - These are larger facilities, sometimes part of an assisted living facility, nursing home or 100% memory care. These types of facilities have less of an at-home feel but often offer more activities and have a wider variety of people to interact with. Most memory care homes or wings are locked to ensure the safety of the residents. They are free to wander within the location, but they won't be able to get out and wander off.

To learn more about options in your area, talk to your doctor, do a search on the internet, and visit different places.

WHAT TO DO NOW...

- Assess the skills and the needs of your loved one.
- Do a safety check of the home and make any changes that will ensure a happy and safe environment.
- Create a plan for care and a plan for relief for the primary caregiver.
- Know where to turn and the support available in your community should you need it.
- Alzheimer's Association 24 hour hotline: 800.272.3900 - put this in your phone in case you need help in a crisis!
- Start researching your options online:
  - www.ElderCare.gov - you can search by zip code and it will give you all the government services and agencies in your area, along with a description of what they do and how they can help. When I put in my zip code there were resources for veterans, help with insurance issues, support groups, counseling and more.
  - www.CareGiver.org
  - www.Alz.org/apps/findus.asp
  - www.APlaceForMom.com
  - www.Care.com

Thinking Through Medical Options

Like it or not, you will have a variety of medical decisions to make in the future. If your loved one understands their diagnosis, talk with them about what they want their care to look like moving forward. If they don't understand, it's up to you and your family to make decisions.

I'm an action taker and a planner. I believe that thinking through some of the what-ifs ahead of time will make things easier when they happen. It is much harder to make a decision, and your choices may be more limited, if you have to figure things out during an emergency or when something is emotionally charged.

There are medical decisions you can say YES or NO to, and there are other things that need to be taken care of. Many of the big Yes/No decisions are covered in legal documents like a living will or the choice to sign a DNR (do not resuscitate - meaning if the person's heart stops, you don't want a medical team to bring your loved one back to life.)

Basic Care Medical Choices

As I'm writing this, my dad has been in a Memory Care Facility for 2 ½ years. I have gotten to know many of the residents and their families and I've supported some through medical emergencies and end of life transitions. How each family handles the medical care of their loved one is different.

Some choose to let nature take its course and only seek medical help or intervention in the event of a fall, broken bone or pain. They discontinue routine care when the disease progresses to a certain point - the point being determined by the family. They feel that when the mind is so far gone, there is no reason to run tests or to give them medication to regulate bodily functions like blood pressure or cholesterol. Instead they focus on comfort measures - is their loved one content, safe and cared for?

Others continue to take their loved one for regular checkups, wanting to know as much as possible about what is going on throughout their body. They want to use every medical option at their disposal to prolong the

Think through care options before you are in an emergency situation. Have a plan in mind.

life of their loved one. They too want them to be comfortable, content, safe and cared for.

Some take extreme measures, others only fix broken bones or things that cause serious pain. There are lots of choices made by families that fall somewhere in between these extremes. There is no right or wrong choice, short of neglect or abuse, just the choice that feels right for each situation.

One thing I also see from time to time, and would like to shine a light on, is the disregard for the choices of others. It is a very stressful time of life for the families coping with the decline of a loved one and making these tough decisions. They know there is no cure, and they don't know how long the journey will last. Emotions run high and many, many people put their opinions and judgements about the proper course of action onto others.

I don't believe people do it maliciously. They believe they are being helpful and supportive. But when someone who has not come to terms with the loss of their own spouse says, "You are so lucky your spouse is still alive!" to someone who is ready for the journey to end, it is anything but helpful. The reverse happens as well. Telling someone they are lucky to be done with the limbo isn't supportive to a grieving family member.

Respect the choices of others.

I have seen and heard of this playing out in support groups too. It's like people go around the room pushing each other's buttons because they believe their choice is the only right choice. The person who chooses to put their loved one in a home advocates for everyone to do the same, saying that their stress levels will go down and things will be a little easier. The person who disagrees with that choice snaps back, "I would never put my wife in a home because I love her." Now the person who put their spouse in a home, who does in fact love them, feels judged and is put on the defensive to justify their decision.

No good comes of that type of exchange. Make the choice that is best for you and your family and respect the choices of others. This is hard enough without turning on and judging each other.

Emergency Medical Care Choices

As people age, balance and judgment decline, the risk of falls, strokes, heart attacks and other emergencies rise. Decide what you want done *BEFORE* the emergency. Do you want first responders and medical professionals to use any means possible to sustain life or do you only want procedures and measures necessary to control bleeding and manage pain?

One day I got a call from my mom that my dad had fallen. They were at Urgent Care and he needed stitches. I dropped everything and headed over, I didn't want my mom to have to deal with it alone, and I wanted to see how my dad was. As they began to stitch up the laceration on his head, the doctor said we needed to take him to the hospital for an MRI. We both looked at her, stunned, and my mom said, "No, I don't want to do that."

The doctor looked back, annoyed, and said, "There could be internal bleeding." She then called for a nurse to be a witness as she told us everything that could happen and how she would not be liable if we chose not to take him. I felt bullied and judged.

My mom explained that my dad had Alzheimer's and began to tear up. He was already a bit confused being in the doctor's office and had adamantly opposed ever having an MRI after the one he'd had a few years before to diagnose the vascular dementia. We didn't see the point of putting him through that procedure when his brain was already impaired, and we wouldn't choose to put him through brain surgery if a problem was found.

The doctor softened, but we still had papers to sign. We had talked about things like this as a family and decided we would do what we could to keep dad safe and pain free but didn't want to take extreme measures, like potential brain surgery. It wasn't easy to say no to medical advice, but it was the right choice for our family.

My dad ended up being fine. He had 11 stitches, which he proceeded to pull out before they were scheduled to be removed. We saw no changes in behavior or noticeable decline in his health.

Know that you have the option and be clear in your convictions and communication if you ever need to exercise them. Think about what you do and don't want done medically before you are in a doctor's office or ER and things start happening without giving you much time to think.

It is really helpful to understand that doctors *not only* have the concern for the patient's well-being, they also need to be aware of their liabilities and potential lawsuits. If you choose to decline their recommendations, there are protocols to cover the legal issues.

End of Life Medical Choices

These are the kinds of questions on a Living Will or Medical Advance Directive - the name of the legal document may vary from state to state. It is good to know what you want to do in these circumstances before a doctor is asking them in a life or death situation.

- Do you want tube feeding if the person cannot eat or swallow on their own?
- Do you want artificial hydration - hydration by means of a tube or syringe if the person can't drink or swallow?
- Do you want blood transfusions?
- Do you want medical treatment that extends life by any means? (Ventilator, etc)

Locational Care Choices

There may come a time when the primary caregiver and their support system can no longer care for your loved one alone. This can happen for a variety of reasons. Some people become violent, confused or paranoid as they decline, and it can be unsafe for the caregiver. Some become so physically unable to do basic tasks like standing up or using the bathroom and the caregiver may not have the physical strength to move and help them. If a person gets out of the house and wanders, you may need more help for safety reasons.

Think ahead about what you want to do so you don't have to make a snap decision in an emergency or under extreme stress. Talk about and explore your options, look at your financial resources and come up with a few solutions. Also talk about where your "lines in the sand" are - what things, if they were to happen, would be cause for a shift in how care was provided.

Here is how things went for my family - every case is different but hopefully hearing our story will make things seem less like a textbook case study and be more helpful to you.

My parents moved to Oregon in September 2012 and the following May we put my dad in a memory care facility. We had no idea things would change so rapidly.

My dad had retired from teaching Astronomy at the university level in 1995. After that, my parents had traveled, volunteered in classrooms, even taught English in China for seven months. When they planned to move to Oregon, my dad decided he was ready to work again. He began reading 900 page books about astronomy "to get up to date". He obsessed over teaching at Reed College in Portland - because his last name was Reed, he thought it was the obvious choice. He wanted me to tell him how to drive there and help him get his resume together.

He also began to contact local schools offering his services as a volunteer in the classroom. I felt terrible and a little embarrassed as I would do a follow up call explaining that my dad was ill and asking them to let him down easy. He was getting very agitated and angry at his lack of success, so we would soften the blow by saying they only have space for volunteers who have children in the school. Our goal was to keep the peace at home, retain his dignity and figure out what to do.

Staying home or running around with my mom was not enough for him and he became more and more focused on finding work and more and more frustrated when he didn't get any. Before Christmas, my sister came out to visit and experiencing the stress of the situation, began a search for options. She found an adult day care nearby and took a tour. She explained the situation to the owner, who came up with the idea of telling my dad he would be a volunteer helping the seniors who spent the day there.

We told my dad we found him a volunteer position and he took it quite seriously. He started off three days a week, always wearing a suit and tie and his name tag, so they would know who he was. He would participate in the activities but was also in charge of holding the door when they would go to another room for lunch, as well as other "duties" the staff found for him. The responsibility and people to talk to helped tremendously and it also gave our mom a break. Her stress levels were very high from trying to occupy and divert my dad all day and then listen to make sure he didn't wander out of the house at night.

While my brother is an actual firefighter, I describe those months my dad lived at home as me being a firefighter as well. I never knew when I would get a frantic call from my mom that my dad had jumped out of the car when it was moving because he didn't like where they were going or that he was doing things in the house and she needed help. On many occasions I had to rush over to intervene. Thankfully I live close and work from home, so I had the flexibility to do what was needed. It was incredibly stressful for all of us.

During this time, we continued to talk to my mom about how things were going and to talk about the what-ifs that were to come. My sister, brother and I were very supportive of her and would tell her that when she couldn't handle it anymore, to let us know, and we would help make whatever arrangements she decided would be best. We looked at some adult foster care homes and a variety of memory care facilities within a half hour of their home. We expected that one day our mom would say "It's time" and we would be able to make plans and transition my dad with as little stress as possible.

It didn't work out that way. Fast forward to Mother's Day 2013. My son came home from college that morning. My son and I, my brother's wife and 3 kids (my brother was working) all went to my mom's for the afternoon to have a family Mother's Day dinner. The minute we arrived I could tell my mom's stress level was through the roof. She and my dad were locked in battle over I can't remember what. My dad, who at the time was obsessed with sweeping the deck and had done it so much that he was ruining the wood, took the twins, now 2 years old, out to sweep with him. My mom began crying and saying how she couldn't handle it.

Shortly before dinner, my dad went off into the green space behind their house with scissors to "get flowers for mom." I vividly remember standing at the kitchen sink with my mom and looking out as he tried to climb over the blackberry bushes. She looked at me and said, "I don't want flowers! I don't want the ones he bought and I don't want the ones he's picking and I'm leaving!" Knowing she shouldn't go alone, I quickly got my shoes and told my 19 year old son, sitting on a stool wide-eyed and not sure what to do, that he had to stay in the house and I'd be back when I could.

My mom and I walked around her neighborhood for about an hour and a half. Her stress level was so high that she has no recollection of it. Looking back, she was probably on the brink of a nervous breakdown, but since I had no experience with them, I didn't know. What I did know was that we had to change the living situation or something bad would happen. That much stress and anger in one house is a recipe for disaster.

> In my family, the kids had to say "It's time to put dad in a memory care home".

That night I got my brother and sister on a conference call and told them what was happening. I said mom is in no condition to make a decision; we have to make it so all she has to do is agree. It's too much for both of them.

I enlisted my husband and his sister to watch my brother's kids the next day. After my mom dropped my dad off at the adult day care, my sister called her to tell her my brother and I were waiting at her house to go look at and decide on a home for dad. I'm not in the military but I imagine this is what executing a shock and awe mission might feel like.

We visited 3 of the homes we had seen before and decided on one. It took a week to get my dad moved in since we needed to get paperwork from his doctor and they had to do a home visit. The home director was willing to continue the volunteer story, knowing that sometimes a white lie was better than an angry outburst. She told my father she had heard how great he was and asked if he would be willing to help her. She told him it would be an overnight position and asked if he'd be willing to do that. He was honored and he said yes. My mom was numb. My siblings and I were stressed and hoped that we could all survive the days until the move was over.

My mom tried to change her mind a few times in the week between Mother's Day and move in day. Hard as it was, I had to resort to tough love and told her we *HAD TO* do this and if she didn't, she shouldn't call me for help the next time something was going wrong.

Adding to the chaos, the move had to happen when my sister and I were in New York City for an annual trade show for my business. My brother decided it would be better for him to facilitate the move during my trip rather than wait until I got back. My husband, son, mom and brother moved things into my dad's room while he was "volunteering" at the adult day care on a Monday. We couldn't take him to the home until Tuesday morning so my mom spent the night with a friend and my brother stayed with my dad. I can only imagine how hard that was and am so grateful my brother was able to do it.

When he and my dad got home, my dad thought the house had been robbed and began to take an inventory. He created a "Things Missing" list. He added questions to the list, "Where are my jeans and sport jackets?" and "Why are the tools and objects in different places from where I placed them?" He also added some notes about the day: "It rained on Monday night."

The next day, my brother dropped him off at the memory care facility where he believed he would be volunteering. My dad realized that his things were there but was never able to piece it together to figure out what had happened.

At about 1 pm in New York, I was in my trade show booth and got a call from my brother. My heart and stomach sank. My sister had left; I knew she was on a bus and couldn't answer the phone. I had to answer to see how it went and to support him. When I heard the pain in his voice I burst into tears and melted to the floor - taking cover behind the table in my booth. That day I learned how very amazing my friends in the art licensing industry were. Without question or hesitation, one came and stood in my booth and others got me to the bathroom so I could pull myself together. They knew this was happening and were ready to help - it was amazing.

My dad tried to call me a few times that afternoon as well, thankfully I had the forethought not to answer while I still needed to be working. When I got back to my room I listened to his messages about being confused and having been robbed. He asked where I was and if could I please come get him. I cried myself to sleep...

I tell you all this detail so you know that the best laid plans often dissolve into chaos. Thankfully we had done some research and knew what care homes we liked the best. Thankfully we were all ready to step up and do what was needed to take care of both of our parents.

This could be how your story plays out, or it could happen very differently. Many people go to a care home from the hospital after a fall, an injury or surgery. Others may have recently wandered and been lost long enough for the family to panic; these families often make the decision for safety reasons. Investigate your options before you are in the eye of the hurricane.

WHAT TO DO NOW...

- Make some choices about basic, emergency and end of life medical care.
- Begin to consider your options and interview people or places to help with care so you are more informed when you need it.
- Talk it out so everyone can get on the same page.
- Keep the needs of your loved one, and the primary caregiver, at the forefront when making decisions.
- Be respectful of differing opinions.
- Be ready to step up and make the tough choices if no one else can, especially if there are safety issues involved.

Notes, Things to Research, Memories and More...

Part 3:
Self Care

"This is the mark of a really admirable man:
steadfastness in the face of trouble."
- Ludwig van Beethoven

If you've ever been on a plane, you know the safety announcements before take-off. Along with showing you how the seatbelt works and where the exits and bathrooms are, they remind you to "put your oxygen mask on first, before helping others." This is excellent advice for life too. Think about self-care as your oxygen mask. If you don't take care of yourself, you won't be much use to others.

Self-care can be a source of guilt for caregivers or family members of people with a long term illness. Many feel they need to feel sad every day to prove their love. They feel guilty taking time for themselves and having fun, knowing that their loved one is slowly slipping away.

Don't push PAUSE on your life.

You can't push PAUSE on your life; it isn't what your loved one would want you to do. You need to live, love and find ways to be happy through this journey - you don't know how long it will last. My dad wouldn't want my family to be upset 24/7 for years - he always wanted us to follow our dreams, seize opportunities and be happy. He lost his brother and both of his parents by the time he was 14 so he fully knew and understood the need to take advantage of the time we have on this earth. He would want that for us now.

It's ok to have duality of emotion. It's ok to...

- be happy when grieving.
- be healthy when someone else is not.
- laugh.

- cry.
- take care of yourself.
- ask for help.
- give and receive support.

Don't beat yourself up about what you *should* or *shouldn't do* - it rarely leads to productive action or good feelings. Do what feels right to *YOU* and respect that others may make different choices.

When my son was little we participated in a co-op preschool that was part of a college class. The preschool was the "lab" and the parents had to attend a 2 hour class once a month, as well as volunteer in the classroom. The teacher was amazing! Her name was Miss Sheryl and there were several things she said that have stuck with me to this day. The one that is relevant to caring for our loved ones and caring for ourselves goes as follows. She was telling us to give up the desire to be "perfect parents" because no matter what we did, our kids will tell us, at some point, that we did something wrong. She said that when that happened, we were to know in our heart of hearts that we did our best and to tell our children the following, "I did the best I could with the knowledge and skills I had in the moment, and when I could do better, I did."

**You are doing the best you can
in a stressful situation. Be kind to yourself.**

Remember to feel your feelings and don't try to wear a brave face 24/7. It is suggested that you don't cry around your loved one with dementia because it can confuse and upset them, so that is when a brave face is appropriate and recommended. But I can assure you, many a tear has been shed in the lobby or in the car outside of my dad's home. You need to allow yourself to grieve.

What I do recommend that may be new to you is this: always end on a positive note. So if you are angry about what is happening, you need to express your feelings but don't stop there. Add a positive feeling at the end of stating what you are feeling now.

Many people will think or say this, "I'm really angry that my dad has Alzheimer's and we have to go through this."

It is more helpful to you in the long run if you take it a step further, like this, "I'm really angry that my dad has Alzheimer's and we have to go through this but I want to feel peace so I can support him and still live a happy life."

Don't stop on the angry emotion.
End with the good feeling you want to feel.

Your ability to focus on what you do want instead of what you don't want is key. If you only focus on what you lost in the person or the struggles ahead, it will be hard to find peace through the process or support your loved one as best you can. When you focus on what you want (and what is possible), you can take action and feel better. You want the person to be cared for, feel supported and be content. You want to ease their pain and yours as well. Make sure what you say you want is something that is possible, or you won't get the results you are looking for. Saying you want to turn back time, cure the incurable, and other things that are impossible is the same as focusing on the pain.

Be Gentle with your Friends

You will find different friends will be willing and able to give different types of support. Learn what they can offer and be ok with it. You will have some friends who don't like to deal with the messy things in life; they won't be the people to call when you need someone to listen when you cry. They will be perfect when you need an escape, a happy outing or a day when you won't be asked how everything is going.

Other friends will be helpful and supportive from a distance. They will be able to have fun or console you depending on your needs but may not feel comfortable with in-person support for your loved one. They aren't the ones to call to stay with your loved one while you leave to do errands or take a break.

Know which friends to go to in different situations.

Still others will be able to do whatever you need to have done. They will be on the phone when you need someone to listen, they will sit with your loved one so you can have a break or they will come with you to look at care facilities. They will be there if you want help figuring out end-of-life arrangements and be just as willing to run off to Disneyland for some fun.

Just as it is hard for you, your loved one's dementia will trigger your friends and family in different ways too. Be aware, ask questions and be ok with whatever they can offer. You need all kinds of support in your life so knowing who to turn to in different situations will be incredibly helpful.

Create Strategies to Relieve Stress

As I mentioned previously, you will get suggestions and well-meaning advice from others that on some days, will push your buttons. If you share your journey as I have on social media, you may trigger others and they may lash out at you.

I once had someone tell me it was shameful that I would show a photo of my father in a "state of decline". She said she would be ashamed if her daughters ever did the same. I obviously triggered something in her and she would go in the "can't handle the messy side of life" friend category had I known her other than online. While I knew her comments were a reflection of what was going on for her, it still stung. I got an instant adrenalin rush and questioned whether I had truly done anything disrespectful in regard to my father. I also cried. In the end I knew it had nothing to do with me, told her that if, heaven forbid, she was ever suffering from Alzheimer's she would be lucky if her children cared for her as much as I care for my father. I then unfriended and blocked her because I don't need that kind of negativity coming at me.

I know there are people that believe I am wrong in sharing my story and what my father and family are going through. By sharing it, I am opening myself up to feedback so I need to be prepared to see it for what it is and not let it hurt me. I know that for every judgment that comes my way I receive the thanks of many others. Thanks for helping them understand, for helping them navigate the disease with their family or for keeping them informed about how my dad is doing. I share my stories and the things I have learned while navigating Alzheimer's - for myself and for those looking for help or understanding. There is no shame in this disease and I believe that my dad, a lifelong learner and teacher, would be glad that something positive can come from his illness.

What do you do when life pushes your buttons? How do you manage long-term stress? Have you ever thought about it or made a plan? Just like every home or building should have a plan in case of an emergency or fire, you should have a plan to help you cope and recover from negative emotions.

> What do you do when life pushes your buttons?

Growing up, one of our family jokes was about my dad and our dog. Whenever things got a little emotional, my dad would pop up and announce that he needed to take the dog for a walk. If I called home from college crying, especially if it was about a boy, he would say, "Wait a minute, I'll get your mother!" and be off the line before I could say another word. He would remove himself from stressful situations when things were happening that he wasn't prepared to deal with. It is socially acceptable to take the dog for a walk or to call on a mother to ease a daughter's pain. I can only assume that this break gave him the time and space to process his feelings before coming back. It probably also saved us all from some unhelpful gut reactions.

Some people go running, for a walk or to the gym. These are temporary escapes, that because of the physical activity involved, also increase stress-relieving hormones. That is why exercise is always mentioned when people are talking about ways to deal with and decrease stress.

I often meditate, listen to calming music or call a friend when I find my stress levels getting too high. Other times I go for a walk or go to a store, a change of scenery and environment can often help. Closing your eyes and taking deep breaths is a great way to quickly bring down your blood pressure and stress levels. Deep breathing is a great tool you can use at a moment's notice, no matter where you are.

Schedule activities that help you manage stress and increase joy into your life regularly. Putting things on the calendar helps ensure you don't fall into the trap of neglecting your own self-care. Massages, therapy, support groups, acupuncture, book clubs, knitting groups, volunteering - these are all great ways to keep joy in your life.

WHAT TO DO NOW...

- Make a list of things that you like to do to keep your stress levels at bay.
- Make a list of things that make you happy - include things that are quick, things that are free and things that might take money and planning.
- Schedule at least one thing off your list every week and make sure you follow through - you are worth it!
- Think about your friends and family and how and when they will be able to best support you. Talk to at least one and ask for the help you need.
- Make self-care a priority so you can be the best caregiver you can be!

Notes, Things to Research, Memories and More...

Part 4:
Connecting with Your Loved One with Dementia or Alzheimer's

"The giving of love is an education in itself."
- Eleanor Roosevelt

THE THREE STAGES OF ALZHEIMER'S

Alzheimer's is divided into three main stages - mild, moderate and severe. The changes in the brain have begun long before symptoms are noticed and a person can be classified into one of these three categories. Symptoms will also vary from person to person. As the doctor once told my family, "If you've met one person with Alzheimer's, you've met one person with Alzheimer's."

Mild Alzheimer's

During the mild stage, symptoms are starting to become noticeable but many may still question whether it's age or dementia / Alzheimer's. Memory issues may become more common - forgetting names, getting confused, misplacing items. The person can usually still function independently, but with more difficulty. Friends and family will likely notice a difference in the person that may not be obvious to people they just met or who don't know them well.

Moderate Alzheimer's

Moderate Alzheimer's is usually the longest stage of the disease and can last for years. It can (in my opinion) be some of the most frustrating times for the person with Alzheimer's. Memory continues to erode and they may begin to forget parts of their life. Mood and personality changes may become more extreme - anger, sadness, paranoia - as they struggle to survive. Changes in sleep patterns may occur and some people begin to have problems with incontinence (bladder and/or bowel control).

As a person moves from moderate to severe Alzheimer's they will begin to need more help with daily activities like dressing and eating. They are also at increased risk of getting lost or having safety issues because of diminished judgment.

Severe Alzheimer's

Severe Alzheimer's is often the hardest on the family but a little easier on the person. They become so lost in the disease that they are usually unaware there is a problem. There is rarely physical pain associated with Alzheimer's (something I cling to as a silver lining). People will become more withdrawn, may stop talking, and they may lose the ability to walk, eat or communicate.

People with severe Alzheimer's usually need round the clock care.

Get more detailed information about the stages of Alzheimer's: www.alz.org/alzheimers_disease_stages_of_alzheimers.asp

JUMP INTO THEIR REALITY

When my dad was first officially diagnosed, my parents had moved to Oregon, and we were beginning to see a lot of changes in him. We went to several meetings about what to expect next.

One piece of advice that has been incredibly helpful was this: "Jump into their reality."

People with dementia and Alzheimer's have minds that seem to be able to teleport. One moment they are in the present and the next they think it's 10 years earlier. There is *NOTHING* you can do to convince them otherwise, until something in their brain shifts again.

This is so important to understand and a big pivot of perspective for friends and family. My dad was a very intelligent man; he liked logic and was the king of reason. Suddenly logic was gone and facts were no longer relevant. He didn't know night from day, he didn't believe that a business was closed just because the doors were locked and the lights were out. If he thought it was daytime, it was.

After he went into the Memory Care Home, I began to experience more of these time-warp conversations with other residents too. I'll admit it was a little alarming at first, but over time I've found them to be some of the most endearing conversations. When you truly join them in their reality, they are happy and you can engage. It's almost like having a tea party with a little girl... but it's not.

Here are a few examples of what I mean so you can see how you might jump in too when faced with this sort of reality confusion.

My day as a government official...

One day I was sitting with my dad - he was mesmerized by a mail order catalog and I had my iPad and my sketchbook open - doing some work. A woman came up to us, very determined, and sat down at the table.

"Are you from the government?" she asked as she grabbed my pen and paper.

"No, I'm his daughter." I replied. This was before I had much experience with jumping into their reality, but it didn't matter, she disregarded my answer anyway.

"OK, I'm going to write my name down." she said. "I need to get out of here. This place is no good and I need you to get me on a bus back to Canada."

My eyes were wide with amazement as I watched her slowly write her name in perfect 1950's cursive. I began to realize there was no convincing her I wasn't with the government.

As she finished her name, she paused. Then said, "I can't remember my address. Oh well - you will know, you are from the government. Please get me out of here."

Then, looking at what she wrote, she got up and walked away with a satisfied look on her face. She never asked me where her bus was because she forgot the whole thing almost instantly. Every time

I see this sweet woman she introduces herself and asks my name as if we have never met. This has been our routine for over 2 years. Each time, I tell her how nice it is to meet her and then I pay her a compliment - I tell her she looks beautiful or notice that she's just had her hair or nails done. Her face lights up and she thanks me. It's a little thing that brings joy to her life and I'm happy to do it!

Planetary Guide...

During another visit with my dad, a woman, who was obviously confused and distressed, stood up from another table. Close to tears, she said, "I don't know what to do now." There was no one nearby to help her so I went and placed her walker in front of her. She looked at me with a confused expression on her face and said, "It's like I've woken up on a different planet and I don't know what to do!"

Those words pierced my heart — this is probably how many of the residents feel, they just can't find the words. As hard as it is to watch my father go through this mental and physical decline, I can't imagine what it would feel like to "wake up on a different planet and not know what to do."

I smiled at her and said, "Well I hope you like it here, I think this planet is pretty cool! Where would you like to go?" We had begun slowly moving forward, in the direction of her room, so I asked if she'd like to go there. As we approached the door she looked at me for confirmation and said, "Is this my room? What do I do now?"

I helped her get into her lounge chair and gave her a book. She seemed content, at least for the moment. Moments are sometimes all we have, and if I can help my father or any of the residents find their way to find peace for a moment, I feel I've done my part.

Car trouble...

It's always interesting when new residents arrive because they are usually the most verbal and also have the most interesting understanding of reality. At least three men I've met believe they built and own the property - although none of them did. On this particular day, my dad and I were looking through a magazine when a gentleman came up behind my dad and touched his shoulder. He then looked at me and said, "I'm sorry to interrupt but I really need to ask him a question."

He then turned to my dad and said, "Will you help me?" My dad replied, "Yes, what do you need?" (This surprised me because he was at the point that his responses rarely made sense so I was thrilled!)

"Do you know where they parked my car?" he asked.

"Car?" my dad said... he was losing interest and turned back to the magazine.

The man continued, talking to me again, "When I find my car I need help fixing it, and I think your dad will know how. I'm going to go look for it, can you keep him here?"

Now I was a little amused because my dad was anything BUT a person who could fix cars. I smiled and told him, "Of course! Let me know if you find the car and we will help you." He walked off, determined.

A few minutes later he came back by the table and introduced himself. It seems the search for the car was forgotten, a new reality unfolding in his mind.

Comparison is the Thief of Joy - Especially in the Case of Dementia

"Comparison is the thief of joy." - Theodore Roosevelt

The quote applies to all sorts of things: work, success, money, houses... it's sort of like the warning to not try to keep up with the Jones' but to instead focus on, and be happy with what you have.

"Comparison is the thief of joy" is particularly relevant when you are dealing with dementia and Alzheimer's. My goal is to find ways to feel as good as I can and help my dad and family do the same. If I start comparing how he is on any given day to how he was when I was growing up, tears immediately come to the surface. The comparison is too sad and devastating. That doesn't mean it doesn't happen - sometimes the comparisons just pop into your head. The key is to notice when it is

happening as quickly as possible and then make the choice to release the comparisons.

"But how do you do that?" I've been asked on more than one occasion. What I do is stop and literally say to myself, "Stop comparing who he is now with the healthy person you remember. It isn't helpful to anyone." Then I begin to look for something to be thankful for in that exact moment. Is my dad content? That makes me happy. Can I help someone or make someone smile? That makes me happy. Can I make my dad laugh or roll his eyes at me? That makes me really happy. I remember that I'm thankful that he has a nice, safe place to live where the staff cares about him. I'm thankful that my parents saved and have the money to pay for it. I'm thankful that it is close to my house so It is easy to stop by when I want to. Change your focus and stop comparing to what was. You will decrease your stress and sadness.

My dad went into the Memory Care Home with moderate Alzheimer's and is now in the severe stage. There are days when he doesn't speak and just stares blankly when you talk to him. Other days he says a few words; he may make or mimic facial expressions or sometimes he gives a quick laugh. Some days he can't remember how to stand up or what to do with a fork. Other days he can move himself but always needs some help. The brain is a complex thing. There are times when he is more connected and aware than others. At some point I assume he will become so severe that he will stop communicating or reacting all together. Instead of thinking about what an accomplished public speaker he used to be, I am now thrilled when he can put 3 or 4 words together that make sense. For my dad today, that is a big win and I focus on and celebrate these small victories.

Remember there are things you can and can't control about dementia and Alzheimer's, and it is futile to waste your energy and effort fighting to change the unchangeable.

Here are some things you can't change:

- You can't change that your loved one has the disease.
- You can't change when or how they will die. After watching a few people I came to care about in the home pass away slowly, with gasps of breath, blank stares and the help of hospice care to manage any pain, I don't want that for my dad. I want him to go peacefully in his sleep. I know, however, that I don't get to decide, but I will be there and be strong however and whenever it happens.
- You can't control the progression of the disease. Every person will go down a different path with different moods, behaviors and time frames. I know people who want the disease to progress quickly and others who want to keep their loved one alive, whether they know who they are or not. We don't get to make those choices.

Here are some things you can control:

- You can decide how you look at the situation. What you focus on will have a huge impact on how hard the journey is for you. Find things to be happy about in the moment and try not to compare your loved one to how they were in the past.
- Hold their hand and hug them. People feel connection through physical touch, just as babies need to be held and loved, so do people at the other end of life's journey.
- Talk to them - you don't know what they can and can't understand so tell them about your day, how you feel, what's going on. They may absorb some and it can be therapeutic for you.
- If they are not living with you, listen to your heart about how often and how long to visit - don't be pressured by the expectations of others. Do what's right for you.

Asking Your Loved One Questions

It is helpful to get in the habit of telling your loved one about simple things they may not know. When I visit my dad I say, "Hi dad, it's me Tara, your daughter." It gives him my name and context and alleviates potential stress and confusion on his part and hurt feelings on my part. Some days he says, "I know" and other days he just looks at me blankly, the explained connection obviously not registering.

I've read and been told that you shouldn't ask someone with dementia questions like "Do you know my name" or "do you remember..." - I'm going to go out on a limb and say I don't totally agree. If you stay in tune to how they are reacting to the questions and stop if they get stressed, then I think its ok. Don't argue or act shocked if they remember incorrectly. Be ok with their answers and if you need to, discuss it with others when you aren't with them. Have a poker face to hide your reactions if you decide to ask questions to see what they do and don't remember on any given day.

When my dad was first in the home, I would ask him a lot of questions to learn more about his childhood or what he was thinking about, knowing his memories would be lost. I had read that typically recent or short-term memories go first but early memories can be recalled longer. I know this was true with my great aunt who I would visit when I was in high school. If we talked about present day events, she would start asking the same questions or giving the same information within 3 minutes. If we started talking about her childhood or young adult life, she could tell me detailed stories for an hour or so.

I assumed it would be the same with my dad, but it wasn't. He had holes in his memory from every part of his life. Was it because his childhood was filled with loss and trauma and he didn't want to remember? Remember, he lost his brother and both parents by the time he was 14. Or was it that his brain was dying in different spots where both his long-term and short-term memories were stored?

I wanted to learn as much as I could - about his life and about how he understood what was happening now. Had I taken the advice of "Don't ask questions" at face value, there are things I wouldn't know today.

While it was very sad, it was also interesting to see how his understanding of who he was had changed. In the beginning he knew he had been a college professor, writer and speaker. That he had a wife, three kids and five grandchildren. Later, when asked if he was married, he sometimes replied with a quick "no". Other times he said he was divorced... he was never divorced. My parents have been married for

> If you are going to ask questions, be prepared for any answer and don't react negatively or in a way that will make the person feel bad about him or herself.

over 50 years. Another time he told me he had 30 children. (Thankfully that is not true! That would be too many siblings for me to keep track of.) At one point he said he had never worked. Through gentle questioning, and stopping if he seemed bothered by it, we could see the changes occurring on more than just behavioral and motor skill levels.

Tell your loved one stories to help them remember or to help you focus on better times - stop if it upsets them or you.

The Sandwich Generation

I am a reluctant member of the "Sandwich Generation"... no, it's not a bunch of baloney - or bologna. It is a term that describes the stage in life when you are still raising your own children and begin to help aging parents. You become the support for both ends of the spectrum - the young trying to figure things out and the older, also trying to figure things out and wondering what on earth happened.

> You are a member of the "Sandwich Generation" if you are still raising children and helping aging parents.

It can be trying and tricky. Fortunately I have both parents and only one has dementia. I know people who have both parents with cognitive issues and that becomes a whole other thing to manage. In our case, while my mom has been incredibly stressed and sometimes needs help making the tough choices, she is willing and able to do what needs to be done.

If you are in a situation where both parents are suffering from dementia or where you have only one parent who is having trouble, you need to get the legal issues sorted out asap so there is someone who can pay bills and make decisions. If it isn't worked out in time, your state will likely get involved; usually not a family's first choice.

As a daughter with one parent with Alzheimer's and one parent without, I sometimes feel caught between supporting my mom and my dad as well as dealing with my own emotions. It feels harder to get support - most support groups are made up of and geared toward the primary caregiver, often the spouse. As a "strong secondary caregiver" - a title I made up - there isn't an obvious place for me. I don't want to go to support groups that my mom goes to and talk about how hard it can be trying to support both her and my dad. I want her to have the space to speak freely about everything going on, even if it's related to me. (Honestly knowing that she will read this makes me uncomfortable, even though we've talked about this!) So where is my space?

What has worked for me has been a more informal support system. My sister lives 3,000 miles away so she isn't able to be an "on the ground" support system. Early on we made a deal, I am here, willing and able to carry much of the load. Her part is to be my phone support. She is ready and willing to talk to me when I need to unload emotions, talk through difficult visits, trying conversations and more. I have a few friends I can turn to. I also get acupuncture regularly to relieve stress. If you are a member of the sandwich generation as well and find yourself in a similar situation, make a plan to get the support you need too.

There have definitely been times when I had to assume the lead role in our family. When my mom has been struggling, I've had to step up and step in.

It happened the Mother's Day when I realized things were really bad, and we needed to move my dad and move him quickly. Other times have been less dire and could often be resolved with humor and hugs - followed by a call to my sister!

One such event took place in my mom's kitchen. My mom had been going to a 6 week caregivers class offered by the county and was getting overwhelmed by all the statistics and decisions that she had to make. Life was moving too quickly and felt overwhelming. It was shortly after my dad was moved and we were all adjusting to the change. My dad was angry and planning his escape from the home. He was asking to leave every time we visited which made us feel guilty, even though we knew we had done the right thing.

I don't remember the beginning of the conversation as my mom and I stood at the counter, cleaning up after dinner, but I remember the emotion. My mom is a spunky, petite half Italian, half Irish woman. She turned to me and said, "In my meeting they say 65% of caregivers die first..." dramatic pause... stomp of foot and then, *"HE'S KILLING ME!!!"*

As she began to cry, it was all I could do not to burst out laughing at the drama of her delivery. I managed to simply smile, wrap her in my arms and say, "Oh mom! When have you ever been in the bottom 65% of ANYTHING! You are an overachiever so I'm sure you will get through this alive."

Thankfully what I said broke the tension and she began to laugh too and didn't choose to grab a frying pan and hit me! It's one of our favorite stories to relive when things get a little heavy. Finding the humor and being able to laugh at ourselves has been a key ingredient to our survival!

I'm not sure where the 65% came from or if it is accurate. When I did an internet search I found a wide range of estimates from 30% and up. Depression and anxiety are regularly cited as an issue for caregivers - usually saying one or both affects more than 50% of caregivers. Keep that in mind and be on the lookout in case a caregiving parent needs extra attention or medical support to help with the ongoing stress.

Notes, Things to Research, Memories and More...

Part 5:
Choosing In-Home Care
or a Care Facility

"Nothing has more strength than dire necessity."
- Euripides

The decision to put your loved one in a care home or to keep them at home and bring in help will be a very personal one. Whether you choose in home help or to put your loved one in a care home, you need to be an advocate for your loved one. The further they slip into the disease the less they will be able to make their wishes and needs known.

Where to provide care as needs increase is an emotional and personal decision.

Bringing care into your home will depend on your financial resources, how you feel about having people in your space 24/7 and how well you can deal with living that intimately with the progression of the disease.

I know a family who made the choice to keep their mother, who suffered from Alzheimer's, at home until the end. They brought in outside help, hospital beds and other mobility devices they needed as the disease progressed. It worked because their mom didn't need as much interaction with others and social stimulus as my dad did. They would read to her, take her to church, watch television and eat together. Siblings would take turns giving the daughter living with the mom breaks during certain days and sometimes for a weekend.

When we were deciding between in-home care and memory care homes, a few benefits of care homes stood out and we ultimately decided that was the way to go for our dad.

How and Why My Family Chose a Care Home

- **First,** he needed more social interaction than he would get if he stayed at home with just my mom and a caregiver.

- **Second,** he was angry at home and resented what he felt was my mom trying to control him for no reason. There were plenty of reasons, many of them safety related, but from his perspective, she was just bossing him around. It was becoming volatile and wasn't worth the risks of a blow up. When people with dementia get angry they can sometimes become violent without notice - even if they have never been violent before the illness. We needed to consider the safety and stress for both of our parents.

- **Third,** my dad was becoming a night wanderer. My mom wasn't getting any sleep and was always worried he would leave the house and get lost in a neighborhood and state they had just moved to. Having a safe and locked environment where he was free to roam in protected areas at all hours was a great solution and stress reliever.

- **Fourth,** the staff at one of the homes we toured pointed out that they would take over the duties of caregiving, safety, feeding, help with bathing and more. We could then resume the role of loving family members. We didn't have to argue with my dad about whether he should shower or whether he should stay inside at 2 am. The conflicts would be greatly reduced, and we could just love him and leave the hard stuff to the care home.

Choosing In-Home Care

If you decide that bringing help into your home is the best option, begin by deciding what type of help you need. Your needs will change as the disease progresses so reevaluate every few months.

- How much and what kind of help do you need in your home?
- Do you need help during the day or do you also need help at night?
- Do you need skilled medical professionals or help with things around the house?

Create a list similar to creating a job posting, because you are going to hire someone or a service that can meet your needs.

Once you know what you need, look for services and options in your area. Ask for referrals from your doctor, local support agencies, friends and people in support groups. Interview until you feel you have found a good fit.

Since you will be bringing someone into your home, be sure background checks have been done, either by you if you will be hiring someone directly or by the agency if you go through a service. You want to feel secure with anyone in your home, and you want to be safeguarded if things were missing.

Choosing a Care Facility

If you decide that care outside of your home is the best choice for your family and loved one, look at several options and decide what fits your budget and what place meets your needs. Talk to the staff, talk to family members with loved ones in the home. Look for reviews online. Explain what you are looking for and see if the information and answers you get feel good.

One way I decided on my first choice was by the environment. Some of the homes we looked at were covered in floral wallpaper and doilies or felt like a hospital ward. They didn't look like anywhere my parents had ever lived, so they didn't feel like the right fit for my dad. It may sound superficial but I wanted the home to feel like a home he would have chosen.

Location was also a factor. The home we chose for my dad is 3 miles from my house and about 4 from my mom's. Having it close makes it easier to stop in more regularly for shorter visits than it would be if we had to drive 30 minutes or more each way. Since we don't know how long he will be there, having a convenient location is helpful.

When touring homes, ask about their payment options. Some will take Medicare or Medicaid right away; others require that you have the money to pay for care for a certain amount of time before they will take Medicare. Medicare rules and qualifications are something to discuss with an elder law attorney.

Connect with Caregivers in Care Homes

While it is up to you to decide how often and how long you visit, it is important to visit so you are aware of what is going on in the home and help you build relationships with the staff. While staff may change several times during your loved one's stay, be nice to the caregivers and talk to them all. It is amazing what you will learn from each one! Also know that when they form a connection with you, they might take a little extra interest in your loved one. Of course they should give equal care to everyone, but they are human and form relationships just like everyone else.

I have seen people scream at caregivers and also complain constantly and berate the service at a home. There may be a merited concern but no one who is caring for those who can't care for themselves deserves to be yelled at on the job. If there is a problem, first decide what you want to happen and what outcome you would like to see. Once you know what you want to see change, be very clear and calm when expressing your concerns to the care home director. Seek resolutions and not just blaming others - your results will be easier and better. Don't take your stress out on the home, it won't help anyone and won't make you feel better!

"Relationships" in Care Homes

One of my first introductions to Alzheimer's was on the TV show, Grey's Anatomy. If you don't watch it, the main character's mother, once a brilliant surgeon, had Alzheimer's and had no idea who her daughter was. Later Chief Webber's wife was also diagnosed with Alzheimer's. During her decline, we saw how she reverted to thinking she was a young girl and later had a boyfriend in her care home. She had no recollection of ever being married. Her husband, Chief Webber had to deal with his wife forgetting their entire life together and learn to accept what was real for her now.

Unfortunately, that storyline is not pure fiction. Many spouses are faced with the same tragic reality. They not only lose their spouse but watch as they form relationships with other residents in memory care facilities. It doesn't always happen and sometimes they are very short lived, but it is good to know that it might happen and prepare yourself in case it does.

When my dad first went into the home, he was quite a catch! Many people wondered why he was there or they thought he was a visitor. The home had to put signs on the doors for a few months warning people that "some of the residents look like staff so if you don't personally know someone, please don't let them out".

One woman had a habit of becoming attached to any new man who moved in. She seemed to mark her territory and be next to him at every meal and ask him to "help her" get to activities. "Help" meant she would grab his arm or hold his hand. You can imagine how odd that was, to walk in and see my dad holding another woman's hand. I can only imagine what my mom felt the first time she saw it!

My dad quickly became a part of a group - he and three other ladies - who would eat together, go to activities and plan their escape. Sometimes they would share their plans with me and I would just listen and nod my head. One that stands out involved them all going out into the courtyard at a specific time, my dad helping one lady get up and over the fence. She would then come around and open the gate and let the rest out. They would then go to the bus stop and then their separate ways. One would go home and another to a friend's house. I believe my dad was going to go to the airport and get on the next plane that would leave the country. He had traveled all his life so for him, it made sense. Thankfully they never actually tried to execute the plan, but I bet they spent hours talking about it!

We talked about it as a family and decided to let it be. My dad thought he had to hold her hand because he thought it was his job as "a volunteer". (I asked and that's what he told me.) We also realized it was helping him adapt to his new surroundings to have a group of ladies who wanted to talk with him, eat with him and plan their escape. We realized he wasn't "cheating" on my mom. He was just doing his best to adapt to a changing landscape.

Other times it can be more than holding hands. I've heard of people becoming very sexualized- making out with other residents and probably more. If you encounter situations like this with your loved one, decide how you want it handled and talk with the care home director. While they can't control every second of a resident's day, they can be on the lookout for couples going into rooms together and work to keep them in common areas. Also understand that your loved one doesn't think they are doing anything wrong and may be very motivated to spend time with this person. Assume that everyone will do their best until the disease in one or both parties progresses to the point of shifting the relationship. If it becomes too upsetting, see if your loved one can be moved to a different area to decrease contact and interaction. My dad's home has two distinct sides to the facility and often a resident is moved from one to the other for a variety of reasons - including inappropriate relationships that are causing undue stress on the family.

Notes, Things to Research, Memories and More...

Part 6:
End of Life Planning

"Tears are the silent language of grief."
- Voltaire

End of Life Plans

Being the planner that I am, it always amazes me when someone dies and there is no plan in place. Not only is the family filled with grief at the death of their loved one after watching them decline, they now have to make quick decisions about what to do next. Do they want a funeral or memorial? Do they want to donate the body or brain for research?

Planning ahead or ignoring the inevitable will not affect the timing or the outcome. I believe it is easier to make plans ahead of time, so you have fewer decisions to make when you just want to grieve.

Here are some things to consider, organize and then save until the time comes:

- Who needs to be notified right away?
- Do you want to donate your loved one's brain and/or body to research?
- Do you want a brain autopsy to have a definitive diagnosis and which can help with Alzheimer's and dementia research?
- Do you have a plan for burial or cremation?
- Will you have a service or other gathering for people to remember your loved one and pay their respects? What do you want that to look like and where do you want it to be?

It can be helpful to discuss a plan of action with your family as well - who will be in charge of phone calls, arrangements, etc. Sometimes you have a lot of warning before your loved one dies and other times it happens quickly. Be prepared.

Understanding Hospice Services & Options

Hospice care is designed to provide comfort care with dignity and respect. Hospice offers extra support to the patient and the entire family when curative measures have been exhausted and the life prognosis is six months or less.

Discuss care options with your Primary Care Physician and when your doctor believes it is time, he or she will make a formal request to the hospice agency of your choice. The agency will meet with you to go over the details about qualifying and to complete any paperwork needed to authorize the hospice agency to provide services and bill Medicare or private insurance. If your loved one doesn't qualify right away, talk to the agency about how to have them reevaluated at a later time.

Before my dad was diagnosed with Alzheimer's, I thought hospice was an absolute indication that death was near. I know many people think the same thing so many families and terminally ill people resist using, or even considering hospice. Now that I have learned more, I think it is a valuable resource that you should take advantage of when your loved one qualifies. Hospice gives extra attention and care for your loved one, helps manage pain and provides support for the family when life expectancy is six months or less.

Some people go on and off hospice several times. They may qualify but then have an improvement in their health and prognosis and then be taken off hospice. If they decline again, they could re-qualify. Going on hospice doesn't necessarily mean the end of life is imminent.

Do your research and talk to people who have used hospice services in the past. If your loved one is in a care facility, find out which programs they like the best and why. The family gets to choose what service they want to use, and it can be quite competitive with multiple options. Take some time to look at your options so you will know who you trust when the time comes.

Remember, as well, that hospice workers are human and not all knowing. It is up to you to be your loved ones advocate and ask questions when you are unsure about treatment or pain management. I have seen hospice be incredibly helpful, and I have seen hospice drop the ball causing a person to suffer more pain than was necessary. If something doesn't seem right, especially if your loved one is in pain, speak up.

Learn more about Hospice...

www.HospiceFoundation.org
alz.org/care/alzheimers-dementia-hospice.asp

In Closing...

As I finish writing this book, my dad is 76 years old and lives in a Memory Care Facility. He has been there for 2 ½ years and is well cared for. He seems content and I visit him often. There are days when he says nothing, and days I can tell he is more aware of what is going on. I have no idea how long our journey will last or how it will end. I don't get to decide the how or the when, but I do get to decide how I show up for him, for my family and for everyone else I encounter who is going through a similar experience.

This book has been a labor of love that required many tissues to write. I thank my family, again, for being open to my sharing so many of our personal stories. I hope you find some comfort in knowing what you can do now to ease your burden moving forward. Making the tough decisions outside of emotional stress make things just a little bit easier.

Sending you strength, compassion and love for what lies ahead...

If Alzheimer's Could Speak...

One night as I was flying home from an inspiring personal development event, I sat on the plane thinking about my dad. I thought about all the things my family has been through up until now and I wondered how the rest of the journey would play out. I began to contemplate what he would say to us – and to my mother in particular – if he could still communicate his feelings. My dad was a firm believer in living life to the fullest, and never putting off until tomorrow what you could do today. He believed in having fun, balancing work and play, and enjoying the days we are given.

I wrote this poem, *If Alzheimer's Could Speak...* looking out of the window of an airplane at the world below. This is what I imagine my dad would tell us – and you – about how to live when someone you love has Alzheimer's.

See a video version of the poem and get a free copy to download and print at PivotToHappy.com/alz-poem

---

"You gain strength, courage, and confidence by every experience in which you really stop to look fear in the face. You must do the things which you think you cannot do."

– Eleanor Roosevelt

If Alzheimer's Could Speak...
by Tara Reed

Talk to me... I can hear your words
and they still touch my soul.

Smile at me... My eyes can see you and feel your
heart even if I don't remember how to smile back.

Hold my hand... I can feel your energy
when our hands connect.
It makes me feel safe and less alone.

Love me... My heart can feel your love
even if my words can't express mine.

Live your life... Help me on my path
but don't press pause on your life.
Be the vibrant person I know and love.

Trust the process...

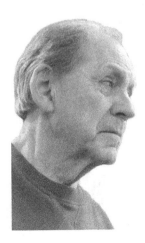

I know this is hard and not
what we planned but
trust the process.
We can't control it but
we can choose our focus.
Remember the good times,
know that I am ok and
that you are in my heart always.

DEC 0 3 2019

9 780692 567623